P9-DTV-595

HUMANISTIC PERSPECTIVES IN MEDICAL ETHICS

Edited by Maurice B. Visscher, M.D.

Prometheus Books, Buffalo
Pemberton Books, London

Prometheus Books - 923 Kensington, Buffalo, N.Y.
ISBN 0-87975-012-X

Pemberton Books - 88 Islington High St. London
SBN 301 73031 8

Printed in the United States of America

Acknowledgments
Aided by a grant to support the work of the Editor by the Louis W. and Maud Hill Family Foundation.
"The Evolution of the Right-to-Health Concept in the United States," by Carleton B. Chapman and John M. Talmadge, was originally published in THE PHAROS, January 1971, and is reprinted by permission.
"Beyond Atrocity: A Personal Psychiatric View," by Robert Jay Lifton, is the introduction to *Crimes of War*, Robert Jay Lifton, Richard Falk, and Gabriel Kolko, editors. Copyright © 1971 by Education-Action Conference on American Crimes of War in Vietnam. Reprinted by permission of Random House, Inc.

The following articles appeared originally in THE HUMANIST and are reprinted by permission: "The Right to Die: Experiences of Two-Thirds of a Century," by Walter C. Alvarez, September/October, 1971; "Birth Defects: The Ethical Problem," by Leroy Augenstein, September/October, 1968; "Prison Doctors: Ethical Problems for Physicians in Relation to Criminal Justice," by Tom Murton, May/June, 1971.

Library of Congress
Catalog Card No: 72-90475
Second Printing, 1973

CONTENTS

EDITOR'S PREFACE

Maurice B. Visscher

Anyone dealing with the problems of deciding what is good is necessarily confronted with age-old questions: good for what, good for whom, and good for when? One also has to deal with competing "goods" when there is no simple dichotomy available for choice.

Physicians living and working today face many ethical questions which were not recognized a generation ago or were not as important as they are now. The mores of the past provide no valid guide to the solution of moral questions in changed contexts. Only a fresh approach from basic principles in the light of current realities can yield answers that promise useful conclusions. By following custom one can avoid criticism for one's behavior, but this has no relevance to ethics. It was once customary to burn some types of psychotics at the stake as witches; religious dissenters were treated in the same way. Enlightenment and the discrediting of once widely held superstitions have now made such practices repugnant to society. One may legitimately wonder whether the currently accepted mores for dealing with persons addicted to the use of psychotropic drugs are not as outmoded as the burning of witches. Our treatment of such persons as felons is not quite as inhumane as burning at the stake, but 10 years or more in a penitentiary is hardly a pleasant experience or a humane treatment for a malady.

Any addition to the literature on medical ethics requires justification. The present volume of essays is presented because no existing treatment covers the realm of problems which late 20th-century developments have brought to the fore. This volume by no means exhausts the field of current problems in medical ethics; it does, however, attempt to deal with the historical and philosophic background for some of the more important practical present-day problems. In recent years there have been important changes in common thought about many ethical concepts. Malthus foresaw the coming of gross overpopulation, but only recently have the grave consequences of the population explosion begun to influence common thinking about the ethics of reproductive behavior. Sterilization, contraception, abortion, and euthanasia have very different kinds of social and individual significance than they did in the simpler days when there were new continents to fill and before technological advance made the pollution of the environment, both local and general, a threat to human health and happiness and even to human survival.

Medical advance itself has changed the ethical frame in which man must now operate. The right to die with dignity to avoid an intolerable existence has become a much more acute problem since modern medicine has acquired its armamentarium of antibiotics, resuscitation devices, and various other life-sustaining procedures. Pneumonia is no longer "the old man's friend," and temporary renal shutdown can be tided over by dialysis. Cardiac arrest can often be corrected, and respiratory arrest can be treated by mechanical artificial breathing for days, months, or even years. Consequently the case for euthanasia has become much more solid. Decisions as to "when to pull out the tubes," or "when to shut off the respirator," or whether to continue antibiotic therapy, or even when and whether to increase the dose of morphine in hopeless and painful situations, have become so frequent that the physician is no longer able to say with equanimity that his single duty is to prolong life as much as possible. The Vatican has recently said that it is not the physician's duty to employ extreme measures to prolong distressful life.

The lowering of the death rate and lengthening of the average life span by control of infectious disease has been the major factor in the current and future population. On the other hand, developments in contraceptive methodology and improvements in the safety of sterilization and abortion procedures have opened new possibilities for control of the birth rate which make older and more simplistic ethical dicta about reproductive behavior questionable or obsolete. Changes in the life style of large segments of our populations have also made it necessary to take new looks at older ethical principles about sexual and reproductive behavior. Monogamous sex ethics can no longer be so heavily reinforced by fears of unwanted pregnancies, because they can be prevented or terminated. No longer is fear of venereal disease the effective deterrent that it once was (despite the fact that such disease is on the rise again). People generally know that the antibiotics have greatly altered the prognosis in such disease states.

The ethics of abortion is a different matter now, given the social danger of overpopulation, than it was when there was no worldwide problem of too many mouths to feed. The personal problem of an unwanted child of promiscuous parents is now more than a personal problem—it has obvious social importance.

Questions regarding the ethics of medical research procedures are very important today, primarily because in our era scientific study of human disease has become so productive of useful results. Percival laid down some precepts about testing therapeutic innovations on patients, but in his time there were not—as there are today—large numbers of physicians whose main professional objective was to increase scientific medical knowledge. Furthermore, until a relatively few years ago the technology for scientific study was comparatively primitive. Only within the last half century has the rise in knowledge of physiology, biochemistry, pharmacology, microbiology and other basic sciences provided the ground upon which clinical investigation could build successfully. Thus although physicians with exploring minds have engaged in what might be called investigation on their patients since ancient times, the magnitude of the effort was insignificant until recently. The avenues open for real scientific investigation were extremely limited. Numerous drugs of plant and animal origin were tested and some valuable agents were found, usually as a result of trying various folk remedies, as in the case of digitalis, derived from foxglove. Opium and its derivatives, cocaine, and quinine were in the same category, as were some drugs from plants indigenous to the Orient such as ephedrine and reserpine, which have only recently come into use in Western countries. The physician played a very small innovative investigative role in these instances. The exploratory observations were made by "herb doctors" or even by total laymen.

Today, however, the sciences of pharmacology and pharmaceutical chemistry are so far advanced that many thousands of new compounds with therapeutic potential are synthesized every year. As a result, their toxicity, mutagenicity and possible efficacy must be tested in numerous ways.

Today exhaustive tests are always made first on lower animals before the drugs are given to humans—except for accidents like the discovery of the hallucinogenic properties of LSD. An organic chemist who produced the chemical inadvertently inhaled some of the airborne powder while he was transferring it from one receptacle to another, and noted shortly thereafter that he had remarkable visual hallucinations. His curiosity was aroused, and after a day or two he purposely ingested a few millionths of a gram of the same powder and reproduced the effect. It should be added however, that the subsequent real scientific study of LSD has involved thousands of animal experiments.

In dealing with the ethical problems of drug testing one meets with a curious phenomenon, namely the rise of a cult of zoophilia which maintains that it is unethical to sacrifice lower animal life in studies of potential new drugs for human use. It is hard to understand the thought processes of people who raise no audible objection to the annual sacrifice of literally billions of lower animals for human food, but scream loudly about the sacrifice of many fewer animals' lives in the scientific study of new drugs and in other types of medical research.

The antivivisection movement is kept alive by a small minority of the human race. Nevertheless, by distortion of the facts it is able to recruit support on specific issues from a much larger fraction of people active in animal humane movements, especially the growing group of dog and cat devotees. For example, by playing on the sentimental attachment of many persons to their personal pet dogs and/or cats, it was possible to obtain laws prohibiting the use of unclaimed impounded animals for scientific study in the whole of Britain and in several states in the United States, Pennsylvania for one. Strenuous efforts are currently being made in other states to accomplish the same end. Medical research is more expensive in states or countries with such laws, and supplies of animals are harder to obtain, even at higher prices.

The ethical aspects of the scientific use of lower animals are therefore of importance to medical scientists as well as to the public at large. This is not a new ethical problem, but it is more important today than before because the medical research enterprise is much larger and especially because future human welfare will be so much determined by whether we can obtain knowledge basic to the control of such diseases as cancer and arteriosclerosis. The list of potentially controllable diseases comprises the whole spectrum of ills to which humanity is heir.

The roles of the physician in modern society are complex and multifaceted. Physicians can play a large role in the humane administration of justice. Many physicians quite understandably shun participation in forensic medical activities, either civil or criminal. Those who do participate are subject to pressures and temptations to slant their reports, or even to falsify findings for monetary or other gains. Fortunately many resist these pressures—for example, the physician who performed autopsies on the victims of the recent Attica prison tragedy and reported findings contradicting prison officials' reports of what had happened. Although physicians engaged in forensic medicine should be, like Caesar's wife, above suspicion, unfortunately they do not always perform in such a way. An unfortunate example, important because of the person involved and the grave consequences of the medical report, was that of the military medical officer who performed the autopsy on the body of John F. Kennedy after his assassination. This officer admitted that he burned his original autopsy notes in his residence fireplace some hours after he had performed the autopsy, and after he had met with government agents, who might very plausibly have had reasons for wanting the autopsy report to support some official views as to the character and probable origin of the late President's fatal wounds. One does not destroy original scientific records without some reason. The hasty destruction of the Kennedy autopsy records leaves a residue of suspicion, both about the motive and about the reliability of the final report, which will be difficult or impossible to erase. The ethics of the autopsy surgeon cannot but be called into question, even if his motive for burning the records were simply to protect himself from a charge of incompetence.

Medical experts who do assume roles in legal matters, civil and criminal, need a high sense of moral responsibility. Society cannot tolerate anything less than complete candor from medical as well as other varieties of scientific experts. This is true not only in connection with personal criminal violence, but equally or more so in connection with other fields. One thinks of scientific studies of environmental pollution, of food and drugs, and of the protection of the public against fraudulent claims for all kinds of manufactured appliances, from automobiles to television receivers.

Physicians have special competence in many areas of social importance, from abortion and drug addiction to the psychiatric effects of military combat. The increasing tendency to view competent medical practice as necessarily dealing with the whole person, not simply with his damaged liver, heart, eyes, spleen, stomach, or kidneys, means that physicians must deal with ethical problems in relation to social situations.

A member of a learned profession has implied obligations to society beyond the honesty and altruism which one expects, or at least hopes, will be exhibited by all men. In addition, one expects or hopes that members of the medical profession will recall that the root meaning of the title "doctor" is actually "teacher." There is, or should be, a *noblesse oblige* attached to the privilege of higher professional education; it includes an obligation to serve society as informed and unbiased experts and "teachers." The American medical profession has been notably delinquent in this regard in relation to habit-forming drug use, particularly in education of the public about humane and effective treatment of drug addicts.

The medical profession has not been totally silent in this regard but it has certainly not been effective in educating the larger public. A broader view of medical ethics would result in the recognition by physicians that they have an obligation to society to educate the larger public about the scientific facts on psychotropic drug addiction and the resulting conclusions concerning appropriate social action.

Contemporary society has in general adopted an egalitarian ethic toward access to health care. The concept of medical care as a right, rather than a privilege of the affluent, has far-reaching implications for medical ethics. The practice of medicine in the United States, and in most other nonsocialist countries, has been based upon a fee-for-service compensation system. Obviously, without some universal total insurance system for the less affluent, such a method of compensation for service is incompatible with the ethic of medical care as a basic human right because the indigent simply cannot pay the costs. In fact, only the very affluent members of society are able to bear the costs of catastrophic illness without great family hardship.

The medical profession today is confronted with a dilemma. The overall cost of health care in the United States has risen almost astronomically along with the institution of Medicare and Medicaid and the great rise in private insurance coverage for professional services and hospital care, paid on an indemnity basis. The costs now exceed 7 per cent of the Gross National Product, and the fraction is rising. In the recent past the fee-for-service system has allowed economically ambitious practitioners to obtain large, sometimes very large, incomes. Any other feasible system of compensation would unquestionably limit incomes. Society at large puts a high value on competent medical care, but physicians are undoubtedly justified in their fear that under a system of socialized medicine their monetary rewards would be apt to decline, relative to other personal compensation in our society. They see that despite the high value placed upon education in modern times, the economic rewards of teachers are not great, not only for primary and secondary school instructors, but for college and university professors as well. They are also justifiably afraid that in a large bureaucracy constraints would be placed upon their professional freedom of decision and action in the care of a particular patient. The farther one works from a source of authority in an organization the harder it becomes to bend or break general rules which may be inappropriate in particular instances. Professional autonomy at the level of the individual physician becomes less possible as the system in which the physician works becomes larger. Thus the advantages to the patient of freedom from economic constraints have to be balanced against the possible losses in professional autonomy and other disadvantages. The physician is therefore not acting wholly out of self-interest when he resists steps toward eliminating the fee-for-service system of compensation. The compelling reasons for substituting some other system are partly economic because the social ethic of equal access of rich and poor alike to high-quality health service cannot be achieved unless it is made economically feasible both for society and for the individual.

The physician plays the key role in determining how much hospital facilities are used. The costs of hospitalization constitute a major fraction of all health-care expenses. Unnecessary use to suit the physician's convenience or the patient's preference is incompatible with economy. Mechanisms for control, compatible with quality medical care, are indispensible if ideal care is to be achieved. As in the case of many other problems, balance must be achieved between one objective and another. Total autonomy of individual professional entrepreneurs is incompatible with larger social objectives.

It is useful to look at the ethical problems of physicians today and at what they are likely to be tomorrow, in the light of history and of philosophy as well as in relation to the changing social scene. This collection of essays attempts to present the thinking of knowledgeable experts in those contexts. Ethics is an evolving set of concepts. There are some fundamental assumptions, presuppositions in other words, about which people must agree in order to discuss ethical problems usefully. The basic presupposition on which the authors of these essays agree is that an improvement in the human condition must be the desired goal. This humanistic orientation is not new to medical ethics, but human welfare is defined differently now from in earlier times, and the role of medical expertise in society has broadened. With the advance of science and technology has come an expectation that all men should be able to share the fruits of those developments in all fields, including medicine.

Hopefully these essays may assist in defining ethical goals for physicians.

CHAPTER 1

THE HUMANISTIC TRADITION IN THE HEALTH PROFESSIONS

THE BACKGROUND OF MEDICAL ETHICS

Chauncey D. Leake

Prehistory

From the earliest beginnings the various health professions have obviously been concerned with the care of sick people. This means giving sympathy and tender care, gaining the confidence of the sick person, comforting and protecting him, seeing to it that he gets appropriate food and is kept clean and free from irritation and annoyance.

The earliest of the health professions was probably nursing. The nurses were presumably the older and more experienced individuals in a family or tribe who had sufficient kindliness and sympathy to take care of those who were injured in accidents or fighting, or who came down with those mysterious illnesses which we now call infectious or metabolic diseases. These nurses would gradually develop confidence in what they were doing, and would gain the respect and trust of their patients. They might have exchanged experiences and developed an oral tradition. When some kind of notation was possible, either by pictograph or scratches on clay tablets, records could be kept. Those older persons who had intellectual capacity could then classify the records, analyze them, and gradually develop concepts about disease and methods of handling it. These would have been the physicians of their day.

Meanwhile, some persons in the family or tribe must have became skilled at identifying plant, animal, or mineral materials that could be used for food or medicine. In this search they must have tried nearly everything. Some materials would have been found to produce purgation, sweating, or even vomiting. Bland, gummy substances might have been found to relieve irritation on the skin. In this way a knowledge of drugs developed, and those who were skilled in identifying these materials, gathering them, preserving them, and preparing them for use became what we would call the pharmacists.

It is important to remember that it was always necessary to take care of the domesticated animals. Veterinary medicine was undoubtedly one of the oldest of the health professions. Various specialties developed as the static cultures arose in China, India, Sumeria, Egypt and even in Middle America. In all cases, however, the members of the various health groups kept their humane purpose in mind: to try to make the sick comfortable and to get them well.

The Attitudes of Members of the Health Professions In Ancient and Medieval Times

In all the great static cultures, early writings attest to the need for decorum in those who would take care of the sick. The early Hindu writings are particularly impressive in this regard. Such people were expected to be clean in their persons, to keep their hair trimmed and their clothes in good order. They were even admonished to keep their fingernails clean. They were urged to approach patients respectfully with gentleness and dignity. They were expected to maintain their skills and to transmit their specialized knowledge by precept and example to younger people who would succeed them.

This humanistic tradition had its practical aspects. In the beginning, it was important for the members of the family or the tribe to be cared for and to be kept in as good physical condition as possible in order to survive. Later on this concept was extended to community groups and even to national groups. Furthermore, payment of healers was frequently associated with their competence in their professional duties. Under these circumstances the members of the health professions acquired very early a social position that was in itself satisfying and rewarding.

Physicians and their helpers must have realized very early that they could help patients by promoting hope, courage, and trust. The early Greek physicians realized that sick people tend to get well if they are given nothing beyond gentle and tender loving care. This was later expressed in the Latin phrase *vix medicatrix naturae,* the "healing power of nature." Although we rediscover this characteristic of illness every once in a while in a very scientific manner and call it the "placebo effect," actually this concept is of extreme antiquity.

The earliest nurses and others who took care of sick people in the small tribes which were commonplace all over the earth had religious connections and often acted as priests. This association of the religious spirit with the healing skill tended to reinforce the overall humanistic attitude expected of the members of the health professions. The precepts established by the early Hindu writers pervaded the known world and became particularly influential in Asia Minor with the rise of the Greek temples of Aesklepios. Here, as in the earlier temples of Imhotep in Egypt, there was a direct association between the priests and the healers who were directly in charge of the care of the sick.

In the Greek world the various Aesklepia became extremely important and deeply respected. They reached their highest development at such places as Kos, Knidos, Epidaurus, Pergamon, Corinth and Athens. The temple was usually built near a spring to provide for clear wholesome water. The regimen was usually a relatively simple one, involving the "temple sleep," in which the incoming patient was probably given wine or beer with hemp or some other sleep-producing agent. During the light sleep the priest and probably the physician would visit the patient and outline a general regimen to be followed. In addition to drugs, diet, or surgery as indicated, this would include rest, bathing, gymnastics, reading and entertainment, including games and dramatic performances or dances. Thus the Aesklepia became cultural centers with elaborate baths, gymnasia, libraries, race tracks, and superb amphitheaters for dramatic productions. A great effort was made to promote mental repose and comfort. Diet was particularly well controlled, with much attention being paid to rounded nutrition adjusted to individual needs.

One of the great Greek centers for health teaching was at Kos, where the renowned Hippocratic school developed. While Hippocrates (460-370 B.C.) was the best known teacher of this group, it is not likely that he wrote all of the many books ascribed to the school. (A delightful fictional account of Hippocrates, *The Torch,* has been published by that great neurosurgeon Wilder Penfield of Montreal.) Hippocrates was renowned, not only for his technical skill and ability as a great physician, but also for his humanistic attitude.

The technical writings of the Hippocratic school are impressive in their rationality. For example, the treatise *On the Sacred Disease* (epilepsy), states directly that the so-called sacred disease is no more sacred than any other, but has a natural cause and will be found to have a natural method of therapy. It has taken a long while to make this faith come true! The rationality of the Hippocratic group is further exemplified in the various books on acute and chronic diseases, on airs, waters and places, on fractures and on prognostics.

Equally impressive are the Hippocratic school's general philosophical writings. The very first of the *Aphorisms* expresses the philosophical calm expected of the physician: "Art is long, life is short, experience deceptive, and judgment fallacious." The attitude of the school is presented more formally in the writings entitled *Oath, Law, Precepts,* and *Decorum*. The famed *Oath,* which is still taken in modified form by graduates of medical schools all over the world, is really an indenture given by young men coming into the group to follow its traditions. Its high moral standards are expressed in a practical manner, in admonitions to preserve the dignity and privacy of the patient. *Decorum* is interesting because it carries forward the general ideas of etiquette which had been so carefully outlined by the Hindu physicians.

The great ancient tradition became extremely influential. It was reinforced during Roman times particularly by the writings of Galen (131-201 A.D.), and was maintained in the magnificent Moslem culture by such writers as Al-Ruhāwī, probably of the ninth century A.D. As far as we know, his *Adab al-tabib* ("the practical conduct of physicians") is the earliest Moslem treatise to deal with medical etiquette and the moral problems facing physicians. He quotes Aristotle and Hippocrates, and applies the three tenets of Galen's *On the Passions of the Soul:* (1) seeking the Aristotelian means of moderation and temperance; (2) freeing the soul from passion by training and practice; and (3) promoting a sound and healthy temperament in the body.

Al-Ruhāwī insists that the spiritual health of a patient is of prime importance, and that its care is a function of physicians. He advises physicians, for the sake of mercy, to maintain silence about the diagnosis in cases of patients who may not understand, and not to discourage any complaints by patients, since they may reveal matters that will help in treatment.

The most important portion of Al-Ruhāwī's writing directs the conduct of physicians in their daily lives. He discusses in detail the management of their own bodies: He notes that the physician should cleanse his body, mouth, and teeth, trim his nails, and remove excess hair from the head and face. His clothes should be useful, well made, and attractive. He should chew well when he eats and sip when he drinks. Physicians should not drink in public, run around with women, or occupy themselves with play. They should keep a daily chart of their activities and prepare records on each patient. In regard to fees, Al-Ruhāwī notes that physicians should earn enough for their needs, so that they can afford marriage, proper food, garments, and housing, and so that their children can be taught the art of medicine.

Physicians are exhorted to attend meetings of virtuous and learned men, to remove evil people from their company, and to value good character more than property. Al-Ruhāwī advocates exposing charlatans and maintaining qualifying examinations for the health professions. Nurses should be trained to be kind, rational, skillful, and willing.

While the Hindu, Hippocratic, Galenical and early Moslem deontological writings served to develop self-governance in the health professions, there were certain to be abuses. Society gave early evidence of clear intent to control medical practice effectively. The main purpose of these early regulations was to ensure competence. The earliest are to be found in the Code of Hammurabi, of about 2000 B.C. This important set of laws, promulgated by Hammurabi, was carved on stelae of black granite and erected in various parts of the Assyrian empire. Of the code's many provisions, some 15 relate to the health professions. The principle involved was "an eye for an eye, and a tooth for a tooth." As translated by President Harper of the University of Chicago, the provisions read something like, "If a physician shall treat a man, and that man shall die, then surely the physician shall die also... If a physician shall treat the eye of a man, and the man shall lose the sight thereof, then surely the physician shall lose the sight of his eye." The same ideas were expressed with respect to other parts of the body. This was a tough code; however, members of the health professions soon learned that they could ransom themselves or parts of their bodies by paying appropriate sums for damages to the patients whom they may have injured.

It is interesting to note that in the ancient Code of Hammurabi the retaliatory damages were based upon the presumed value of the life of a physician to himself, or upon the value of any part of his body. This is quite different from the principle in our modern malpractice suits, where the damages are expressed in terms of the value to a patient of his own life, or the part of the body that may have been injured. It would seem that in general physicians may value their own bodies and lives more highly than those of their patients. If modern malpractice lawyers were to take this tack, we might see a further rise in the already enormous sums now sometimes granted in malpractice suits.

Most of the great figures in medicine have emphasized the broad scope of the responsibilities laid upon the members of the health professions. For example, Al-Ruhāwī indicates that physicians are responsible for the conduct of their nurses and must look after the preparation of pharmaceutical remedies if others cannot do so. It is, therefore, essential that physicians have the skill to identify accurately the remedies which they may use and to be able to prepare them effectively for administration. As indicated by Sanci Hamarnek,[2] the Moslem pharmacists held to a high standard of cleanliness, deportment, and skill. The various Moslem communities maintained competence in medical practice by an examination system and the appointment of civil overseers.

The high standards expressed by Al-Ruhāwī were not unusual among the great Moslem physicians. One of the greatest, the Persian Al-Razi (865-925), based his high sense of moral idealism on religious grounds. Well known in our own times is Rabbi Moses ben Maimon, usually called Moses Maimonides (1135-1204), who came from Cordova and was court physician to Saladin. He left an important treatise on personal hygiene involving sound precepts for nutrition, and his *Guide for the Perplexed* is a rational effort to harmonize Aristolelian moderation and temperance with Jewish canonical regulations. Without going into the detail expressed by Al-Ruhāwī, Maimonides nevertheless added his immense prestige to the promotion of general humanistic ideals in regard to effective medical practice.

These admirable precepts were extremely influential as Moslem culture became known to the medieval world. Much of the high standard of personal conduct expected of members of the health professions was transmitted almost without change from the ancient Hindu and Greek sources through Moslem writers into medieval Europe, especially through the trading port of Salerno with its secular medical school. More significantly, there was increasing recognition of the importance of assuring competent medical care. The various Germanic tribes had imposed the provisions of the *lex talionis,* the law of the claw, in regard to individuals who professed skill in the care of sick people. George Fort, in his discussion of medical economy during the Middle Ages, quotes a seventh century Visigothic law which strongly resembles the ancient Babylonian Code of Hammurabi.

The first extensive law relating to medical practice in Europe was established by the great Emperor Frederick II in 1224. This specified the type of instruction that a physician was to receive, required an examination and license to practice, and regulated the fees that might be charged. Furthermore, the law attempted to control public hygiene, to regulate the sale of food and medicines and to prevent adulteration. This law's requirement that anyone desiring to treat the sick for a fee must pass an examination from the physicians in the School of Salerno did much to establish that school's pre-eminence. The significance of Frederick's statute may be judged by the fact that it was re-enacted by Charles IV for the German States in 1347, and established for Italy in 1365. In short, with the rise of the city-states during the later medieval period, the practice of medicine became more and more regulated by local statute.

During the medieval period a distinctly hedonistic note crept into the moral precepts of medical writers, as indicated by Henri de Mondeville in the 14th century. After all, members of the health professions must earn enough for themselves and their families to live decently, this is expected of them. Nonetheless, they were well aware of patients' attitudes toward their payment. Euricius Cordus, the physician-father of the famed Valerius Cordus (1514-1544), who discovered ether, wrote the well-known verse "*Tres Facies Habit Medicus*":

Three faces has the doctor:
A god's when first he's sought;
And then an angel's the cure half wrought;
But when comes due the doctor's fee,
Then Satan looks less terrible than he.

During the Middle Ages the generous idealism of the Greeks was in danger of being forgotten, lost among the meticulous details of professional deportment devised by such scholastics as the Salernitan teacher, Archaimathaeus. Nevertheless, the long-standing nobility and dignity of the health professions were strongly insisted upon by such well-known leaders as Guy de Chauliac (1300-1370), Paracelsus (1493-1541), and Ambroise Paré (1510-1590). A little later in England, the great reputation of Thomas Sydenham (1624-1689) made his inspiring example particularly important in promoting the tradition of wholesome personal honor in medical practice.

As physicians and surgeons formed colleges and guilds during the Renaissance, they became very jealous of their position and powers, and were enabled by their charters to deal with quackery and immoral or unskillful practice. For example, one may note the laws enacted during the reign of Henry VIII of England, at the instigation of what is now the Royal College of Physicians, chartered by Henry in 1518. (This remarkable monarch had already chartered the Barbers-Surgeons Guild in 1512, which forbade the practice of surgery by any except members of the guild, and conferred on them the rights to train new members and to examine applicants for practice.) These early ordinances required high moral standards in the relations of practitioners to their patients, enumerated the reciprocal obligations of members to each other, and indicated the attitude to be taken by the members of the colleges to the public at large.

Turmoil of the Industrial Revolution

The transition from the broad principles of high standards for the health professions to the current complicated system arose during the 18th century—the time of the great Industrial Revolution, when machinery began to supplant craft. People moved from the rural areas, from a basic and long-established agricultural economy, into the slums of the big industrial cities, and the established conventions of centuries were overthrown. The situation was particularly acute in England. In the great mills of new manufacturing centers such as Manchester and Liverpool, the workers were grossly exploited, even children being expected to work 12 hours in a shift. Prices rose, and the poor people had little comfort except to get drunk nightly on cheap gin.

This also was the time of the recognition of the philosophical significance of law and order in nature, as a result of the discoveries of Isaac Newton (1642-1727). People sought to find immutable, detailed, and comprehensive laws for every phase of their activity to match those established mathematically for the movements of the heavenly bodies in the skies. This tendency was reflected—not deliberately, it is true—in the writing of Thomas Percival (1740-1804), who formulated a "Code of Medical Ethics." Given his purpose of covering all possible contingencies in interpersonal relations, two results were certain to follow: a growing emphasis on letter instead of spirit, and a conflict in the multiplicity of rules.

Handicapped physically by poor vision and headaches, Percival was a scholarly and judicious thinker, highly respected for his personal charm and character. He was deeply concerned with the social problems of his time, and did his best to try to correct them. He was born in 1740 in Warrington, Lancashire. His parents having died when he was a youngster, he was brought up by an uncle who was a physician. Thomas Percival was a dissenter and received his medical education in Edinburgh, where he must have come into contact with many of that remarkable group from North America who did so much to shape future medicine in the United States, men like Benjamin Rush (1745-1813) and David Hosack (1769-1835). Percival received the degree of Doctor of Medicine from Leyden in 1765. Here he must have been greatly influenced by the brilliant clinical expositions and high standards of practice in the tradition of the greatest medical teacher Europe ever saw, Herman Boerhaave (1668-1738). Percival settled in Manchester, England, where he conducted a quiet and dignified practice, chiefly as a consultant. He often employed medical apprentices as secretaries and with his friends aided in the establishment of the Manchester Literary and Philosophical Society which did so much to help promote the newly developed experimental sciences in England. Percival attempted to promote general methods of collecting and analyzing vital statistics and to prepare an effective census. With the rise of industrial manufacturing he was deeply impressed with the need for improving factory hygiene; he advocated regulations for ventilation, restrooms, and general cleanliness. He insisted upon the necessity for a board of health with police powers to regulate lodging-houses, tenements, water supplies and sewage disposal.

Percival understood the need to promote satisfactory interpersonal relations between the different kinds of health professionals in England during the latter part of the 18th century. There was much friction among them over their prestige and authority in the new infirmaries established in the major industrial cities in order to take care of the indigent workers. In order to understand the significance of Percival's ethics, it is important to realize the status of the three groups of medical practitioners: physicians, surgeons, and apothecaries. Quite an elaborate system of etiquette existed between these groups, but there was considerable professional jealousy among them.

The physicians generally came from established families and had independent means; they had received the degree Doctor of Medicine from a university. Although they did not have to practice for a livelihood, it was expected that they would, from the kindness of their hearts, advise indigent sick people. They never soiled their hands by operating. Since they did not send bills, it became customary for their patient to leave a gold guinea on the hall-table as he left the home of the physician. This was the origin of the usual internist's fee of five dollars prevalent until a few decades ago!

The surgeons, however, usually had no particular family background or independent means. They did not go to the universities, nor did they receive the degree of Doctor of Medicine. (English surgeons still prefer to be called "Mister.") As a result, they tended to charge their patients whatever the traffic might bear—a tendency surgeons still have. In general, the surgeons in 18th century England had to rely upon the physicians to refer patients to them. Nevertheless, many of them practiced directly, accepting any or all patients who might come to them.

Then there were the apothecaries, who were tradesmen, usually keeping the trade in the family and passing the apothecary shop down through several generations. The apothecaries were the first line of health defense. People would come to them when feeling ill and ask if something could be done for them. Frequently the apothecaries would give them some relatively mild drug, and trust to luck. On the other hand, it was expected that if the apothecary thought the condition was serious, he would refer the patient to a physician.

This relatively rigid caste system among the physicians, surgeons, and apothecaries was bound to result in stiff formality and jealousy. This was greatly intensified when the public hospitals were established in the manufacturing towns, and the physicians, surgeons, and apothecaries strove for positions of prestige in the new clinics and infirmaries. Under these conditions there was bound to be much friction, with resulting loss of adequate health care for the indigent sick people.

Thomas Percival cogitated long and carefully over this matter, and consulted many of his influential friends, not only in Great Britain but also in the United States. He tentatively drew up a "code" to regulate the interrelations of the physicians, surgeons, and apothecaries. He seems to have realized that this was mostly a matter of preserving decent etiquette. Nevertheless, he was unfortunately persuaded to call it a "code of ethics."

Actually, Percival's Code was extremely influential. After circulating among friends for a number of years, it was finally published in 1804, when Percival himself died, and was formally adopted as the code by which the conduct of physicians, surgeons, and apothecaries in the various clinics and infirmaries would be managed. The penalty for failing to conform to the code would be suspension of privileges, or even expulsion from the institution. Percival's Code is actually a sort of Emily Post guidebook for decent interpersonal relations. It has little to do with the serious moral problems facing the health professions.

The Evolution of Medical "Ethics" in the United States

During the first two decades of the 19th century, there was rapid frontier expansion in the United States. Distances were long, and communications poor. It was necessary that the people moving into the frontier area have some kind of medical attention. The result was that medical schools were established in almost every small community in the westward moving areas. Usually these were apprentice schools in which local physicians trained youngsters by direct methods.

Benjamin Rush (1745-1813), in his teaching in Philadelphia, made every effort to instill in his students high principles of conduct and deportment. The first significant medical school established west of the Allegheny Mountains was Transylvania Medical School in Lexington, Kentucky. Here a distinguished faculty was assembled, and some effort was made to promote adequate medical instruction, even though it might only be for a couple of years. Nevertheless, it included dissection, some chemistry, and much *materia medica*. High standards of deportment were stressed. However, the situation in the country generally had become so unsatisfactory by 1820 that it was almost scandalous. Samuel Brown (1769-1830) of Transylvania University thought that he could improve conditions by organizing a secret fraternity of the better physicians—the Kappa Lambda Society of Aesklepios, which tried to promote high standards of personal conduct among the members. The Society formally established Percival's Code as its guideline for conduct. Abridged editions of Percival's work were published in Philadelphia in 1821 and in Lexington in 1822, and were widely circulated among the profession.

The Kappa Lambda Society flourished for a while, establishing chapters in the major cities, but came to grief during the 1830's as a result of the gross hedonism of the New York chapter. The members of this group tried to obtain control of the hospitals, but were generally repudiated by their colleagues.

Nevertheless, a general reforming spirit was under way in the United States. By 1823 the New York State Medical Society had established a "Code of Ethics," and a similar publication was issued in Baltimore in 1832. In both these instances Percival's Code was acknowledged as inspiration. Nonetheless conditions did not greatly improve in the United States. In an effort to improve the poor standards of professional training and conduct, Nathan Smith Davis (1817-1904) succeeded, in spite of opposition, in organizing the American Medical Association in 1846. At its first annual meeting in Philadelphia in 1847 came the formulation of a code of ethics, with the establishment of minimal requirements for medical training.

The American Medical Association Code of Ethics also specifically acknowledged its derivation from Percival.

It gave local, state, and national medical societies the power to suspend or expel members who transgressed any of its provisions. The major obligations as outlined in this book of etiquette were "of the duties of physicians to their patients and of the obligation of patients to their physicians, and of the duties of physicians to each other and to the public, and of the obligations of the public to the profession." There was a certain amount of sweet conceit in all this!

Difficulties arose in the provisions regarding relations between members of the American Medical Association or its constituents, who were presumed to be adequately trained, and those who were thought to be inadequately trained. The difficulty began over consultation with the "homeopaths." These were serious and well-trained individuals who adhered to the rather restricted theoretical position developed by Christian Friedrich Hahnemann (1755-1843). He revived a Paracelsian idea that symptoms of diseases are relieved by the particular drugs that produce effects resembling the symptoms. Homeopaths also thought that the effectiveness of a drug is enhanced by giving it in infinitesimally small doses.

Since many homeopaths were very intelligent and gentle practitioners, they flourished. Actually they were simply rediscovering the ancient Hippocratic principle of *vis medicatrix naturae:* People tend to get well regardless of treatment. There was much popular lay support of the homeopathic idea, but the regular physicians were forbidden by the code to consult with them. So much trouble resulted that the New York Medical Society attempted to revise the code and permit its members some reasonable contact with the homeopaths. At the St. Paul meeting of the American Medical Association in 1882, however, delegates from the New York Society were refused admission.

At the 1883 meeting of the New York State Medical Society, a codified system of conduct for physicians was abandoned entirely. It was proposed instead that the exercise of a right of discipline in a medical society should be extended only to cover those circumstances which are "comprehended under the commission of acts unworthy of a physician and a gentleman." Many of the outstanding American physicians made a careful study of the situation. The conservative group in New York withdrew from the original medical society and organized themselves separately, adopting the code of ethics of the American Medical Association. This ridiculous situation lasted until 1903.

Compromise was reached at the New Orleans meeting of the American Medical Association in 1903 when a report was made by a committee appointed to consider the general problem of conduct of members of the profession. The findings of this committee were not satisfactory to one of its more thoughtful members, the highly respected pathologist at the Johns Hopkins Medical School, William Henry Welch (1850-1934). With astonishing speed, Welch prepared what he thought to be a suitable system of advisory precepts in medical conduct, and had it distributed anonymously to the delegates at the general meeting. His personal influence was great enough to secure its adoption. This then became the "Principle of Ethics" of the American Medical Association and was much more satisfactory than the older "code." The "exclusive dogma" clause was omitted from the section on consultation, and local medical organizations were given the privilege of interpreting the principles of conduct as they might see fit.

Throughout this development the aphoristic style of Percival's original code had been preserved. It has, of course, the fundamental difficulty involved in any rigidly formulated code of conduct. With continual amendment its various provisions tend to become contradictory. Furthermore, it lends itself to authoritarian interpretation, in which the letter of the regulation becomes more important than the spirit of the effort. In general, the medical conservatives like a stiff and rigid code so that those who violate it may be thrown out of the organization, while the more liberal tend to look upon these guidelines as means of inducing members of the health professions to follow reasonable and acceptable social principles of behavior. In 1957 the rules of deportment among members of the medical profession were further simplified when the American Medical Association established 10 general principles to govern the conduct of its members.

Through this long development of Percival's Code and its modifications in the United States, distinguished and respected leaders of the medical profession throughout the world continued to insist upon humanistic values in medical practice. Similar general principles for conduct were established by dentists, pharmacists, nurses, and even veterinarians. Still, in actual practice medical humanism tended to suffer. The competition among physicians, and among the members of the various health professions, caused increasing difficulty in maintaining high standards on behalf of individual sick people, or public welfare as a whole.

As an example, one may note the long continued effort on the part of the American Medical Association to oppose development in various fields of public health. Expansion of public health services was thought to endanger the individual incomes of individual physicians. By the beginning of the 20th century, verifiable knowledge about health and disease had become so advanced that preventive medicine could well be undertaken on a large scale. Indeed, William Henry Welch proposed that every medical school make a basic effort to develop preventive medicine. Although every effort was made by the medical schools to promote the idea, the practicing physicians did not support it. A cynic might suggest that they felt that any success in preventing disease would cut into their own incomes.

What happened is what usually results when an impasse of this sort is reached: The people at large take up the issue. Public health measures were generally enacted by the people themselves, in spite of vigorous opposition from much of the medical profession. The success was so great as to bring totally unexpected problems upon us. By increasing the life span and by cutting down infant mortality, we have increased our numbers all over the earth so that we are reaching toxic levels. We are in each other's way, suffering enormous tension, creating mountainous wastes, and polluting and destroying our environment. Again, these are public problems, and people generally seem to be more aware of them than are most of the members of the health professions, who should be providing the leadership.

The general problem of purposes and motives, and thus of conduct, mood, and behavior, is a question to which many answers have been given over the centuries. These answers comprise the various systems of ethics. On the other hand, the verifiable information that we have about ourselves in health and disease raises the question "What is truth?" To this question also many answers have been attempted over the centuries, and these comprise the various logics. The most satisfactory current logic is that embodied in the scientific method, which permits of independent verification. There then arises the problem of selecting from the vast amount of verifiable information about ourselves in health and disease that which is appropriate and fitting to the particular patient. This calls for judgment. One may be taught the ethics and the logics, but one can only acquire judgment by practice. It is here that the arts and the humanities play a major role in the health professions. Fortunately this is increasingly appreciated, particularly by students, who are recalling the basic Hippocratic principle that medicine is both an art and a science. The science consists of the verifiable information available on health and disease. The art consists in being able to apply this effectively for the benefit of individual patients.

Ethics in the Health Professions

The general distinction between ethics and etiquette to which I had referred in my study of Percival's *Medical Ethics*[3] came into full recognition comparatively recently. The significant difference between basic moral problems and matters of mere etiquette and courtesy were, of course, strikingly apparent in connection with the various atrocities committed by Nazi physicians on prisoners and minority groups during World War II. It was the general world-wide revulsion against these acts which resulted in the Nurenberg Code of Ethics for the health professions, which is simply a modification of the ancient Hippocratic Oath to include interdiction of any experimentation upon human subjects without their consent. This led later to the Helsinki declaration and then to the Geneva form of the Hippocratic Oath which was adopted by the United Nations and is in general use throughout the world.

A systematic analysis of basic moral, and thus ethical, problems associated with the health professions was recently undertaken by Joseph Fletcher, the brilliant theologian of Cambridge Theological Seminary. His study *Morals and Medicine*[4] raised those sticky problems which the members of the health professions have usually tried to avoid. These concern abortion, contraception, euthanasia, the right of a patient to die, the right of a patient to know the truth, and the specific responsibilities of physicians in connection with genetic deformities. This book has helped to bring such matters into public focus, and it has aided in the modification of social attitudes and laws. Currently, many areas of the world are legalizing abortion, a trend that not only serves the welfare of individual women, but also alleviates population pressures and genetic disturbances. In spite of powerful religious opposition, the general principles of contraception are well accepted socially. This has been aided greatly by technical advances which make contraception a relatively simple matter. Nonetheless, Fletcher's effort did not come to grips with the conflicting ethical theories which have become quite disturbing with more recent technical developments in the health professions, such as those connected with organ transplantation.

The ethical position proposed by Joseph Fletcher has much significance for the health professions. He is developing "situationalism," the belief that careful consideration of the consequences of action, in relation to the situation, may result in the most satisfactory procedure. This, of course, marks the end of any absolutism in ethics, except in the sense of potential ideals. Telling the whole truth is no longer absolutely moral; right action depends upon the situation, and upon the welfare of the various personalities and conditions involved.

If the health professions are to maintain their prestige, it is essential that their members not merely understand the standards of etiquette they are supposed to follow, but also that they appreciate some of our growing difficulties with conflicting ethical theories. People generally are becoming aware of these problems. Humanism remains as a paramount factor in the success of health professional practice. The association of agapic love of the art *(philotechnia)* with love for humanity *(philanthropia)* is quite as pertinent now as it was in Hippocratic times.

References

1. This work has been translated and well analyzed by Martin Levey in *Transactions of the American Philosophical Society,* n.s. 57, Part 3 (1967).

2. *Bulletin of the History of Medicine*, 42 (1968), pp. 450-461.

3. C.D. Leake, *Percival's Medical Ethics* (Baltimore: Williams and Wilkins, 1927).

4. J. F. Fletcher, *Morals and Medicine* (Princeton: Princeton University Press, 1954).

List of Recommended Readings

No bibliography dealing with ethical theories can be presumed to be complete. The following works, arranged alphabetically, are pertinent to the discussion.

E.M. Albert, T.C. Denise, and S.P. Peterfreund, *Great Traditions in* Ethics (New York: American Book Company, 1953), 362 pp.

E.G. Conklin, *The Direction of Human Evolution* (New York: Scribner's, 1921), 256 pp.

———, *Man Real and Ideal* (New York: Scribner's, 1943), 278 pp.

W. Fite, *Individualism* (New York: Columbia University Press, 1911), 333 pp.

———, *The Examined Life* (Bloomington: Indiana University Press, 1957), 345 pp.

J.F. Fletcher, *Morals and Medicine* (Princeton: Princeton University Press, 1954), 276 pp.

———, *Situation Ethics: The New Morality* (Philadelphia: Westminster Press, 1966), 176 pp.

S.R. Graubard, ed., "Symposium on Ethical Aspects of Experimentation with Human Subjects," *Daedalus* XIV, 98, pp. 219-597.

O. Guttentag, "Ethical Problems in Human Experimentation," in Torrey, *Ethical Issues in Medicine* (listed below), pp. 195-226.

C.J. Herrick, *The Evolution of Human Nature* (Austin: University of Texas Press, 1956), 506 pp.

S.J. Holmes, *Life and Morals* (New York: Harper's, 1948), 232 pp.

T.H. Huxley and Julian Huxley, *Touchstone for Ethics* (New York: Harper & Row, 1947), 186 pp.

I. Ladimer and R.W. Newman, eds., *Clinical Investigation in Medicine: Legal, Ethical and Moral Aspects: An Anthology and Bibliography* (Boston: Boston University Law-Medicine Research Institute, 1963), 517 pp.

L. Lasagna, *The Doctor's Dilemmas* (New York: Collier Books, 1963), 352 pp.

C.D. Leake, *Percival's Medical Ethics* (Baltimore: Williams & Wilkins, 1927), 291 pp.

_____, "Ethicogenesis," *Science Monthly*, 60 (1945), pp.245-253.
_____, "Technical Triumphs and Moral Muddles," *Annals of Internal* Medicine, 67, No. 3, Part III (1967).
_____, "Theories of Ethics and Medical Practice," *Journal of the American Medical Association*, 208 (1969), pp. 842-847.
_____, "Ethical Theories and Human Experimentation," *Annals of the New York Academy of Science*, 169, pp. 388-396.
_____ and P. Romanell, *Can We Agree? A Scientist and a Philosopher Argue About Ethics* (Austin: University of Texas Press, 1950), 110 pp.
N. MacDonald, ed., "Symposium on Medical Ethics," *The New* Physician, 18 (1969), pp. 117-136.
M. Otto, *Science and the Moral Life* (New York: Mentor Books, 1954), 210 pp.
E.F. Torrey, ed., *Ethical Issues in Medicine: The Role of the Physician in Today's Society* (Boston: Little, Brown and Co., 1968), 433 pp.
M.B. Visscher, "Medical Research and Ethics," *Journal of the American Medical Association*, 199 (February 29, 1967), pp. 631-636.

CHAPTER 2

MEDICAL ETHICS IN PHILOSOPHICAL PERSPECTIVE

Patrick Romanell

I

Half a century ago, when my friend Chauncey Leake began his pioneer work on the historical background of the ethics of medicine, he regretfully noted in a challenging edition of Thomas Percival's *Medical Ethics* that writers on the subject had "seldom availed themselves of the philosophical analyses of the principles of ethical theory made by recognized ethical scholars."[1] As a result, although certain cases related to medical jurisprudence are discussed in the last chapter of the 18th-century English physician's influential manual, his book is somewhat mistitled because it deals more with the professional rules of medical *etiquette* than with the basic principles of medical *ethics*.

This explains why all the subsequent codes of medical ethics patterned after Percival, including the well-known one adopted by the American Medical Association in 1847 and frequently revised and abridged thereafter, were written without the aid of professional philosophers. No moral philosopher is ever really needed to draw up a fixed set of rules for the professional conduct of physicians and surgeons. All one needs is a medical Emily Post.

Even that most ancient and revered Magna Carta of medical ethics, the Hippocratic Oath is, alas, not altogether free of the element of professional courtesy. It will be recalled that the first provision of the oath has to do with economic and educational matters, and includes the implied stipulation that the sons of a doctor's teacher should receive medical training gratis. Such vested interest in self-perpetuation of the guild should not be too difficult to understand; no code of professional ethics, however idealistic in intent, is going to be so unrealistic as to legislate the profession out of existence and business. After all, as Shaw said, doctors are morally no better (and no worse) than any other group of men, regardless of what the codes of medical ethics may say or imply to the contrary. To believe otherwise is to live under an illusion that can only terminate in disillusion.

There are some rather promising signs at present that the medical profession may at long last be on the verge of going beyond its traditionally ingrained but superficial view of medical ethics as professional etiquette. Both the general public and enlightened spokesmen for the medical profession have recently become concerned with certain crucial medico-ethical issues. These range from the ever active debate between individualized and socialized medicine to widespread concern over all sorts of population, pollution, and "pot" problems, as well as to increasing anxiety over "iatrogenic" disease, human experimentation on the living, and organ transplantation from the dead.

Nevertheless, despite all the current interest in such issues, some theoretical ordering of the pertinent material is needed if we are not to miss the forest for the trees, and if we expect the field itself of medical ethics to come of age philosophically. Keeping this objective in mind, we are first going to suggest an all-inclusive scheme for classifying moral problems generally so that we may be able in due course to spot with greater ease their counterparts in medicine particularly. In the final analysis, the moral problems of medicine are nothing but the moral problems of men writ small. Medical ethics, therefore, must properly be considered a special branch of ethics as a whole. If we learn nothing but the advantage of juxtaposing general and medical ethics instead of keeping them apart as is customary, our whole attempt to bring the moral aspects of medicine into proper philosophical perspective will not have been made in vain.

To begin *in medias res,* the generic trait of any moral problem in life is *conflict.* The rules of conduct and the principles of ethics would be utterly superfluous if we did not experience conflicts over how to live. Now, moral conflict is of necessity bipolar, because it logically takes two poles of opposing value to make a conflict between them possible. But what precisely are the two poles of a moral conflict?

Conventional morality and traditional ethics assume as a self-evident truth that there is only one type of moral conflict whose two poles are *good* and *bad* (or their equivalents). One obvious consequence of this deep-seated assumption is the traditional definition of ethics itself. Another, less obvious consequence is an unwitting but serious gap in practically all the existing literature in ethics: The traditional concept of moral struggle concentrates so much on the problem of evil that it pays no real attention to the more tormenting problem of good in human life.

Ever since the publication of G.E. Moore's *Principia* Ethica (1903) there has been considerable discussion of his miscalled "naturalistic fallacy" in ethics. However, in the heat of all the polemics, scholars have neglected a more common and much more serious instance of reductionistic fallacy—"the rigoristic fallacy," to coin a name for it. While the first fallacy is a technical error in those ethical theories which reduce moral to factual terms, the second fallacy is the traditional mistake stemming from the reduction of the moral itself to right-and-wrong terms *alone.* This oversimplification of the grammar of ethics is reflected implicitly or explicitly in almost all the classical systems of morality. Even John Dewey, who is far from narrow in his whole approach to moral conflict, follows tradition in defining ethics as "the science that deals with conduct, in so far as this is considered as right or wrong, good or bad."[2] Ethics so defined is, at most, only half the story, resting as it does on the unwritten but erroneous assumption that all moral struggles are reducible to a single type.

I first detected the monotypic presupposition of the traditional concept of moral conflict when I started to work on a paper, "A Vision of the Two Americas," prepared for the Third Interamerican Congress of Philosophy at Mexico City in January, 1950 and published in Spanish the same year in the spring issue of a Mexican professional journal. In that paper, which led me eventually to a more comprehensive view of moral struggle and to a redefinition of ethics to fit, I suggested in aesthetic terms a distinction between two irreducible types of conflict in order to account for the underlying differences of life style in Latin America and Anglo-America. On the one hand, I described as *epic* the traditional conflicts between good and evil because every epic is addressed to the overcoming of obstacles to good—that is, to the overcoming of evil in some form or other—and celebrates the ultimate triumph of good. On the other hand, I characterized as *tragic* the subtler conflicts between good and good, because every genuine tragedy represents, not a battle of good against evil, but a clash of two *goods* (or duties) that happen to be incompatible with each other under certain circumstances.[3]

The difference in polarity between a tragic and an epic conflict may now be deduced from the foregoing and stated technically. Whereas in the epic type of conflict one pole enjoys the positive value of good and the other suffers from the negative value of bad, in the tragic type both poles are positive in value; hence the problem of good arises from their mutual incompatibility. Logically speaking, the difference between epic and tragic conflicts as types of moral struggle may be restated as one between antithetic and antinomic situations, respectively. A moral antithesis is a situation in life where there are avoidable conflicts between two possibilities of conduct, one of which is accepted as right, the other as wrong. Hence the possibility of pathetic misconduct, due to wrong choice. A moral antinomy, on the other hand, is a situation in life where there are *unavoidable* conflicts between two possibilities of conduct. They are considered as apparently of equal merit per se, yet one is chosen at the sacrifice of the other. Hence the possibility of tragic misfortune, due to fatal choice.

This implies that life's problem of good is much more serious than its problem of evil. It is easier in principle, if not in practice, to overcome evil than to abandon good, notwithstanding that in a tragic situation the gain of one good inevitably incurs the loss of the other, thus spelling ultimate defeat. (To see concretely in two classical models why the problem of good is greater than the problem of evil, compare the difficulties of the Sophoclean Antigone with those of the Homeric Odysseus.) It also follows that the conflict of right and wrong, which is the primary concern of traditional morality and organized religion, does not exhaust the entire class of moral situations. Therefore, an adequate theory of ethics, to be complete in its coverage of moral questions and relevant to the complexity of life, must not overlook its tragic manifestations, however poignant and disconcerting they may be. Otherwise, for one thing, those who consider a critical variety of humanistic naturalism as the most reliable and viable philosophy for the guidance of mankind will be in no position to meet effectively the most weighty objection of our critics, who accuse the naturalistic ethic of being insensitive to the tragic dimension of life.

In conclusion, there are two pure or absolute types of moral conflict in life: (1) good-versus-bad (the essence of an epic situation), and (2) good-versus-good (the essence of a tragic situation). In addition to these two absolute types, there is a third or relative type of moral conflict, falling in between the other two, namely, better-versus-worse. All these three distinct types of moral conflict are found throughout life, but perhaps appear most clearly in the daily practice of medicine. Having finished our bare outline of the tripartite typology of moral conflicts in human life as a whole—epic, comparative, tragic—we are now ready to show how the conflicts arise for the medical profession.

II

An excellent confirmation that traditional ethics concerns itself primarily with the problem of evil in general and with the right-versus-wrong kind of moral conflict comes from the popular handbook of the A.M.A. entitled *Principles of Medical Ethics*. Apart from the niceties of professional etiquette, the handbook focuses on "malpractice" in the broadest sense (including the legal); that is, on professional misconduct. (Interestingly enough, the medico-legal term *mal*practice conveys the meaning of "bad" or "evil" in its very etymology.) To select a typical example of professional misconduct from the Special Edition of the *Principles*, "fee-splitting" is condemned as "unethical" essentially because it "invites physicians to place the desire for profit above the opportunity to render appropriate medical service."[4]

It is obvious that the A.M.A.'s official condemnation of fee-splitting belongs to the traditional right-versus-wrong species of moral problems, declaring flatly as it does that it is morally wrong for members of the medical profession to put the profit motive above the service motive in their professional life. Carping cynics would be quick to deny that the medical profession actually believes what it preaches (let alone practices it), but that is irrelevant to the point in question. Violations of a moral rule, however frequent, do not necessarily invalidate it, though they cause at least embarrassment to the violators who merely preach it. Besides, out of fairness, it should be added that the A.M.A. has always been quite cognizant of the extensive fee-splitting abuses in the medical world. In fact, its stand on this point is equally firm: "Wide extent of an unethical practice," the A.M.A. has stated categorically, "does not make it ethical. Ethics has to do with principles, not numbers or locality."[5] In other words, moral truth is not determined by counting noses or taking a Gallup Poll. Thus, in theory at least, the A.M.A. is not on the side of ethical relativity, even if it is not on the side of the angels.

On the contrary, the old relativist and the new "situationist" in ethics, whatever their differences, would contend that what is morally right or wrong depends on the particular circumstances. As circumstances vary, so our judgments of right or wrong must vary accordingly. Unfortunately, I cannot enter here into the grand old debate between absolutism and relativism in ethical theory, so may I refer in passing to my brief examination of the subject elsewhere.[6] As regards the current view called "situation ethics," which seems to be a new name for the old utilitarian way of moral thinking delegalized and personalized, suffice it to say for the moment that its motto could well be the proverbial saying: "New circumstances teach new duties." True, but what do we do when new duties for the benefit of each and every person conflict with old ones? Reach a working compromise to fit the situation? Fine, but "compromise" is a political term, strictly speaking, not a moral one.

Whether we are relativists, absolutists, or neither in our general approach to right-versus-wrong questions, there is no easy way out of the daily problems of morality. That this is the brute fact of the case becomes even more clear when we turn to better-versus-worse questions in medical ethics. Better-versus-worse problems are harder to resolve than right-versus-wrong ones in that they require more decision-making. To illustrate, take the question: Is it better or worse for doctors to treat people while they are well, or wait till they get ill? Needless to elaborate, this is not the same kind of question as the one asked by the A.M.A.: Is the solicitation of patients"[7] right or wrong?

Another illustration of the comparative type of moral conflict is given by Karl Menninger in his illuminating foreword to Joseph Fletcher's provocative work *Morals and Medicine:* "If an isolated doctor has 10 patients, with enough serum to save five lives, which five shall he save? Or shall he run the risk of saving none by dividing it equally among them all?"[8] Under the circumstances presented, which is the better thing to do? Even Fletcher, at present a dauntless champion of the "new morality" whose only absolute in his situational ethics is Christian love, would have to think twice before answering.

Although the handbook of the A.M.A. pays considerable attention to right-versus-wrong problems, it pays none to the most perplexing type of problem confronting a medical practitioner. But this is not the fault of the A.M.A. While right-versus-wrong matters of conduct are subject to codification, right-versus-right ones are not and can't be. There are no Ten Commandments for the tragic side of medical life, as every wise doctor knows only too well from daily experience. Because the tragic type of moral conflict has traditionally suffered either neglect or misunderstanding in the literature on medical ethics, the remainder of this essay is devoted to some dramatic instances of it in medical practice.

To return to Menninger's foreword, we have already taken from its first paragraph his example of a better-versus-worse question in medical ethics. Even though he does not stop to make the typological distinction, in the same paragraph he raises two other questions belonging this time to the tragic type of medico-ethical problems: "Suppose the worst man in the world applied to the best surgeon in the world for relief from a condition that would prove fatal unless relieved by surgery. Should the surgeon operate? Suppose a man, while committing a murder, breaks a leg, but escapes immediate capture and applies to a doctor for relief? Should the doctor treat him?"[9] By the way, Dr. Menninger mentions the name of an American physician who was actually sentenced to prison for treating a murderer, but our interest here is in the moral, not the legal, aspects of the case. Morally, the two questions boil down to this: What should a doctor do when, under circumstances beyond his control, he finds himself torn between being a good citizen and a good physician—between two *conflicting duties?*

The very fact that Karl Menninger raises such questions shows his awareness of the doctor's real dilemma, which lies in the tragic problem of good, not in the epic problem of evil. Using a Roycean term, he refers to "the recurring problem of loyalty which arises over and over in the life of every practicing physician. Every doctor has loyalty, we may assume, to certain medical ideals, to certain social ideals, loyalty to the law of the land, loyalty to religious convictions, loyalty to his family. Conflicts in loyalty adherence are inevitable."[10]

This last sentence by one of our profoundest psychiatrists says it all very neatly and compactly, pointing to the agony and tragic plight of every conscientious physician. Menninger does not spell out the tragic import of what he says about life's conflicting interests, but that is the experience of the loyalty problem for any person, physician or otherwise. The most difficult issues in moral and spiritual life belong to this genuinely tragic domain. Proof positive of this is to be found in our next example of euthanasia, which presents perhaps the most distressing problem imaginable to any responsible physician with a sense of compassion. Let us turn to the Hippocratic Oath for a look at this problem of "mercy killing" or "mercy dying" and let us do so despite the oath's implicit injunction against the practice.

Among the several injunctions of the oath, two consecutive ones stand out. They correspond to two duties of the physician which come into conflict under certain conditions. One tells the physician to do everything within his power "for the benefit of the sick" and to "keep them from harm and injustice."[11] (This, of course, is the celebrated first principle of Hippocratic medicine: *Primum non nocere.*) The other forbids the physician to "give a deadly drug to anybody if asked for it," or even to "make a suggestion to this effect."[12] This statement implies that euthanasia is prohibited on the natural ground that it is the duty of a physician to keep the sick alive until the bitter end.

Now, suppose a physician has patients with terminal illnesses or inoperable tumors who are suffering endlessly and needlessly. What exactly is his duty here? If he keeps such patients alive with heroic remedies, he may find that he cannot keep them from harm and suffering. Down if he does, down if he doesn't! Popularly put, this is the essence of any conflict-of-duties situation in life. Joseph Fletcher, good sport that he is, has recently acknowledged that he was "mistaken" in *Morals and* Medicine when he saw that the Hippocratic Oath includes "two promises" of the ideal physician which, when a "patient is in the grip of an agonizing and fatal disease," turn out to be "incompatible"—these being the promise "to relieve suffering," and the promise "to prolong and protect life."[13] But Fletcher was, in truth, correct originally. For in its two major precepts on the duties of a physician the oath reflects precisely the tragic conflict which is inescapable in medical practice and inevitable sooner or later during the course of a professional career. In the existentialist language of Sartre, the title of every tragic situation, in life as in fiction, is *No Exit*.

I should like to end on a happier note by returning to Thomas Percival for a last illustration of tragic conflict in medical practice. As I see it, by far the best thing in his whole manual, *Medical Ethics*, appears not in the text itself, but in one of his notes appended to it. The note is a remarkably judicious commentary on the following statement in the text: The physician should be the minister of hope and comfort to the sick."[14]

Percival's note on this textual statement, which is evidently inspired by the Hippocratic Oath, raises the old question on medical lying that crops up again and again in the literature: Should a physician tell his patients the truth about what ails them? Or should he lie to them? We already know how Kantian ethics, especially, would answer this medico-ethical question: All lying is wrong, *ergo*, medical lying is. Period. How does Percival handle the question of telling the truth in medical diagnosis?

Instead of resting content with the traditional approach to the question as simply an epic struggle on the part of conscience with the forces of temptation, Percival first of all restates the whole problem in its tragic context. "Every practitioner," he discerns, "must find himself occasionally in circumstances of very delicate embarrassment, with respect to the contending obligations of veracity and professional duty."[15] He then proceeds to specify under what special conditions it would not only be morally proper for physicians to tell a lie, but morally improper for them to tell the truth. To state his position *in nuce,* medical lying is not always bad, and similarly, medical truth-telling is not always necessarily good.

Percival, however, is not just being indulgent on the issue, nor is he oblivious of its possible abuses. Rather, he is speaking for all conscientious physicians who do not make exceptions to the moral principle of truthfulness on the grounds of casuistry or face-saving, but do so because they must make a choice between two incompatible duties—telling the truth, on the one hand, and doing no harm, on the other. If they choose the second or professional horn of the dilemma, this in itself does not remove the tragedy of the situation, to be sure; it only leaves its tragic quality in an arrested state for the time being. Even so, once it is understood that *as physicians* they may have to resolve the incompatibility of duties by choosing that course of action judged to be of greater benefit to the sick, we will then appreciate all the more what might be called the doctor's "iatrocentric predicament" in such tragic situations.

To let Percival speak for himself on the moral justification of what I have termed elsewhere "mercy lying,"[16] I quote the following passage from his long note on the subject:[17]

> Moral truth, in a professional view, has two references; one to the party to whom it is delivered, and another to the individual by whom it is uttered. In the first, it is a relative duty, constituting a branch of justice; and may be properly regulated by the divine rule of equity prescribed by our Saviour, to do unto others, as we would, all circumstances duly weighed, they should do unto us. In the second, it is a personal duty, regarding solely the sincerity,

> the purity, and the probity of the physician himself. To a patient, therefore, perhaps the father of a numerous family, or one whose life is of the highest importance to the community, who makes inquiries which, if faithfully answered, might prove fatal to him, it would be a gross and unfeeling wrong to reveal the truth. His right to it is suspended, and even annihilated; because its beneficial nature being reversed, it would be deeply injurious to himself, to his family, and to the public. And he has the strongest claim, from the trust reposed in his physician, as well as from the common principles of humanity, to be guarded against whatever would be detrimental to him. In such a situation, therefore, the only point at issue is, whether the practitioner shall sacrifice that delicate sense of veracity, which is so ornamental to, and indeed forms a characteristic excellence of the virtuous man, to this claim of professional justice and social duty. Under such a painful conflict of obligations, a wise and good man must be governed by those which are the most imperious; and will therefore generously relinquish every consideration, referable only to himself. Let him be careful, however, not to do this, but in cases of real emergency, which happily seldom occur; and to guard his mind sedulously against the injury it may sustain by such violations of the native love of truth.

Wherever we stand with regard to Dr. Percival's humanitarian defense of medical lying, the crucial thing about it for us here is its paramount bearing on the requirements of a comprehensive theory of ethics, medical and general. The Kantian system of morals, which represents an epic theory of ethics at its traditional best, takes the unnecessarily rigid position that all lies are black, on the ground that their motive is presumably always morally bad. But "mercy lying" in medical diagnosis is a clear-cut case which, ironically, conforms to Kant's own principle of the primacy of motive of duty in moral conduct as such. If a sense of duty is the only motive which counts morally, then on the Kantian hypothesis "mercy lying" as a professional duty performed in good faith must be morally worthy, for the simple reason that *some* doctor's lies at least constitute actions done from duty. On Kant's own ground, however, this line of reasoning is negated in advance by his absolute prohibition of lying in the first place. To compound the irony, Kant is acutely perceptive about those peculiar difficulties in intellectual life he himself called "antinomies," and yet he is apparently not perceptive at all about their counterparts in moral life. After all, if man is stuck with irreconcilable truths in metaphysics, he also may be stuck with irreconcilable duties in ethics. In a word, just as our intellectual life has its tragic moments, so does our moral life.

To sum up in closing, the Kantian brand of traditional ethics in particular sees everything so exclusively in right-or-wrong terms that it remains blind to the tragedy and complexity of human life. For this reason "mercy lying" in its eyes is always a contradictory term and can never be an antinomic one, by definition. Consequently, Kant's legalistic point of departure makes no special allowances for *legitimate* deviations from the standard norm, simply because his conception of the good life and a just society does not permit such leeway in principle. As a final thought, let me say that a serious inquiry into various types of moral conflict found within the medical profession will provide an excellent true-to-life laboratory for testing the validity and applicability of our general hypotheses in ethics. This in itself makes the study of medical ethics philosophically respectable and of the greatest relevance to the moral problems of mankind, especially at a critical time like ours when simplistic solutions to them just won't do.

References

1. Chauncey D. Leake, ed., *Percival's Medical Ethics* (Baltimore: Williams & Wilkins, 1927), p. 3.
2. John Dewey and James H. Tufts, *Ethics*, rev. edition (New York: Holt, 1932), p. 3. Cf. p. 174.
3. Patrick Romanell, "Una Visión de las Dos Américas," *Filosofia y Letras*, Vol. XIX, No. 38, April-June 1950, pp. 389-390. English version, in *Making of the Mexican Mind* (Lincoln: University of Nebraska Press, 1952), p. 22. Cf. "Medicine and the Precariousness of Life," *Philosophy Forum*, Vol. 8, No. 2 (December, 1969), pp. 3-34.
4. *Principles of Medical Ethics, Journal of the American Medical Association*, special edition (June 7, 1958), p. 40.
5. *Ibid.*, p. 41.
6. Patrick Romanell, *Toward a Critical Naturalism* (New York: Macmillan, 1958), pp. 69-81.
7. Ref. no. 4, p. 28.
8. Karl Menninger, Foreword, in Joseph Fletcher, *Morals and Medicine* (Princeton: Princeton University Press, 1954), p. vii.
9. *Ibid.*
10. *Ibid.*
11. Cited in Ilza Veith, "Medical Ethics Throughout the Ages," *A.M.A. Archives of Internal Medicine*, Vol. 100 (September 1957), p. 505.
12. *Ibid.*
13. Joseph Fletcher, "Elective Death," in *Ethical Issues in Medicine*, ed., Fuller Torrey (Boston: Little, Brown, 1968), p. 142; *op. cit.* in ref. no. 8, p. 172.
14. Ref. no. 1, p. 91.
15. *Ibid*, pp. 193-194.
16. Patrick Romanell, "*Morals and Medicine: A Critique,*" *The Humanist*, Vol. XVI, No. 1 (January/February 1956), p. 33.
17. Ref. no. 1, pp. 194-195.

CHAPTER 3

THE SANCTITY-OF-LIFE PRINCIPLE

A PHILOSOPHIC BACKGROUND FOR THE CONSIDERATION OF EUTHANASIA

Marvin Kohl

This work was supported in part by a fellowship from the National Institute of Mental Health (1 FO3 MH43718-01). I am also indebted to J. O. Wisdom both for his suggestions and inspiration. The paper was presented at the Third Euthanasia Conference, sponsored by the Euthanasia Educational Fund, The New York Academy of Medicine, December 5, 1970, and at the American Philosophical Association Western Meeting, Chicago, Illinois, May 7, 1971.

In the following paper I wish, first, to analyze different versions of the sanctity-of-life principle and inquire what, if any, justification there is for believing that life is sacred; and second, to point out certain confusions, especially in regard to euthanasia, that appear to be connected with the erroneous notion that one ought never kill an innocent human being.

The analysis which follows does not purport to be exhaustive. I thought it better to make a reasonable case against more viable positions than to spend time refuting weaker ones. Hence I shall have little to say about the killing of animals or the claim that one ought never kill any human being—not because these problems are unimportant, but because I feel that others are more important.

It is often said that "human life is sacred." This sentence is thought to express a "sanctity-of-life principle," or "SLP" for short. That men actually talk this way, that they use the same speech or orthographic patterns, does not mean that they are all saying the same thing, or that the principle is simple. In fact, the opposite is the case. The SLP is open to, and is often given, different interpretations. It is chameleon-like, changing its colors according to the moral theory it rests upon. It is almost as if a family of related but differing principles were hidden under the rubric of the SLP in order to give the impression of moral consensus.

Consider the following sentence-types:

(1) One ought never kill an innocent human being because in some religious or protoreligious sense life is sacred;

(2) One ought never kill an innocent human being because such an action would be unjust;

(3) One ought never kill an innocent human being because such an action may (or must) lead to undesirable consequences; and

(4) The sentence "One ought never kill an innocent human being" expresses an ultimate moral principle.

Generally speaking, Roman Catholic writers[1] emphasize (1), and use (2) and (3) as supporting arguments. Albert Schweitzer[2] and Edward Shils[3] seem to use (1) and (3) as complementaries, and Yale Kamisar[4] and others use (3) to argue against euthanasia legislation. (4) is important because it contains the word "ultimate" the ambiguity of which leads to the muddling of different claims.

Religious and Protoreligious Interpretations

I shall begin with a brief evaluation of traditional theism, then consider Schweitzer's approach, and conclude with Edward Shils' notion of a protoreligious metaphysic.

According to the traditional theist, God is a personal, all-powerful being, a sovereign who rules *over* his creation. Hence:

> Man is merely the custodian of life, not its Master . . . It is man's duty to accept the decisions of God, not to pass judgments on them. If God has created and bestowed life upon man, it does not fall within the right of man to destroy it.[5]

> Man is not absolutely master of his own life and body. He has not *dominum* over it, but holds it in trust for God's purposes.[6]

The difficulty is that if we grant that an all-powerful God has absolute sovereignty over human life, then if He himself held human life to be sacred, i.e., if He really cared, He would interfere. At least, He would cure the sick; at most, He would prevent unjust illness and accident. If He does nothing, we can only conclude that either His sovereignty is limited (meaning perhaps that He wants us to act), or His power is limited, or He simply does not care.

In other words, if God is what the traditional theist says He is, why doesn't He interfere in cases of unjust illness and accident? On the other hand, if God is not what the theist says He is, and does not interfere with nature—i.e., if He does not "play" God—then either He wants us to make decisions and to act, or He does not. If He does not, then He is a nonmoral god—at least, so it would seem to me.

Although this argument may be countered, it is not so easily met. For instance, someone may suggest that the existence of a moral God does not entail the conclusion that has been drawn. He probably would remind us that God is just, distributing happiness among men according to their deserts, but that this distribution essentially occurs after death. Hence from this point of view God is moral, even though it does not always appear so. This counterargument is a variation of an old but ingenious attempt to explain away the existence of evil. But this eschatological explanation will not do: At best it is mere conjecture, and at worst, theological illusion. Moreover, when we examine the concept of morality as it seems to show itself in the words of Jesus and other writers, we observe that benevolence, or love, and related behavior (such as self-sacrifice) are deemed to be necessary conditions. This would seem to indicate that justice in its narrow sense is not a sufficient condition for morality. A just God need be just, but He need not be moral.

One of the merits of Albert Schweitzer's approach to this problem is that he does not presuppose or establish a basic antinomy between God and man. God, as conceived of by Schweitzer, reveals Himself in the world as the mysterious creative Force, but within man He reveals Himself as ethical Will. "All living knowledge of God rests upon this foundation: that we experience Him in our lives as will-to-love."[7]

This maneuver helps avoid the major pitfall in the traditional theistic position. Since God, for Schweitzer, is part of the life force as ethical Will, God "plays" God when man acts ethically. For if I understand Schweitzer correctly, God expresses His sovereignty through man, and shares it with man. When we care, when we are concerned, He is also expressing care and concern.

Since God is in the world, and since He is part of the life force as ethical Will, it is necessarily true that if God is sacred, then life is sacred. And since God is sacred, it follows that life is sacred. Notice the beauty of Schweitzer's argument. All the statements are linguistically true. The logic is impeccable. And most important, it provides the grounds for the credibility of the sanctity-of-life principle.

Unfortunately, however, the argument is factually vacuous. That is to say, the premises are true, but analytic. The sentence "God is in the world" is true because "being in the world" is part of what is meant by the word "God." "God is part of the life force as ethical Will" is true because "being part of the life force as ethical Will" is part of what Schweitzer means by "God." "God is sacred" is true, because by "sacred" is meant "made holy by association with God". And I venture to say that even the most ardent skeptic will admit that if there is a God, it is quite likely that He is in close association with Himself.

If doubt still lurks, if questions remain as to the logical status of the conclusion, then I suggest the following test: Take the statement "life is sacred" in this particular theological context, and see if it can be falsified. See if evidence, even in theory, can be found that would count against its truth. I think one would be hard pressed to find any. Notice that the problem of finding evidence is not merely a practical difficulty, but has an air of logical impossibility about it; for it makes about as much sense to look for empirical evidence to show that "life is sacred" is false, as to look for evidence to show that "seven plus five equals 12" is false.

Edward Shils' notion of a protoreligious metaphysic is plagued by similar difficulties. According to Shils, "the idea of sacredness is generated by the primordial experience of being alive, of experiencing the elemental sensation of vitality and the elemental fear of its extinction."[8] The inviolability of human life is then self-evident, since it is "the most primordial of experiences."[9] But what, may I ask, would count as evidence against this claim? About 200 children die every year from lead poisoning because we are not overly concerned about slum children—would this count as evidence? Again, as many as 400 thousand children may be lead-poisoned, half of them ending up with permanent handicaps[10]—does this count? And what of the *conservative* estimate that as many as 23 thousand traffic fatalities in 1969 resulted from drunk driving? Or that cirrhosis is the sixth leading cause of death? Yet little or no fuss is made over the sale of alcoholic beverages. The American Cancer Society tells us that lung cancer, which has been linked mostly to smoking, will kill more than 51 thousand men in the United States in 1970.[11] More recently, Nicholas Johnson (F.C.C. Commissioner) claimed that "there are 300 thousand deaths a year related to cigarette smoking."[12] Nevertheless, the sale of cigarettes is still legal. If all this (and the surface has just been scratched) does not count against the self-evident status of the inviolability of human life, then what does count?

Shils evidently believes, first, that one must know the truth in order to properly recognize it; second, that those who do not have this prior understanding cannot see the truth, at least not as he conceives it; and third, that the reason people do not have this prior understanding is that they are morally misguided or obviously evil. He grudgingly admits that "there is, in fact, no situation in which the acknowledgment of sanctity-of-life is guaranteed."[13] Nonetheless, he insists on abusing those who would disagree with him, those who do not acknowledge the SLP. In more kindly moments, he dismisses those who do not agree as advocates of "Prometheanism" or the prophets of what he calls "contrived intervention";[14] in a more revealing opening statement, he says that "to persons who are not murderers, concentration camp administrators, or dreamers of sadistic fantasies, the inviolability of human life seems to be so self-evident that it might appear pointless to inquire into it."[15] Evidently Shils believes that two opposing moral interpretations cannot be equally respectable, and that it is therefore necessary to condemn at least one of the interpreters as immoral.

Perhaps Shils was aware of these difficulties, for there is a shift in his position, an attempt to cover the empirical claim under the cloak of a normative one. In the same passage where he maintains that the sacredness of life "is the most primordial of experiences," and that "the fact that many human beings act contrarily, or do not apprehend it, does not impugn the sacredness of life," he goes on to suggest that the proposition in question "is not more than a guiding principle." Surely, if it is no more than a guiding principle, no more than a normative principle, then it is not a natural metaphysic, it is not in the nature of things. If something is the case, then it makes little sense to say that we ought to make it so. If life is really sacred, then it makes little sense to say that it ought to be so treated. On the other hand, if there is nothing in the universe which necessitates or guarantees the sacredness of life, and if the claim is only that life *ought* to be treated as being sacred, then it makes even less sense to argue that there is a protoreligious natural metaphysic. Shils cannot have it both ways.

But some men are reluctant to talk in the first person, and are reluctant to say "I think we ought to treat human beings in such and such a way", or "I think we ought not kill." Instead they prefer to give their desires and preferences an impersonal sense of importance. Hence, we are told that cosmic forces, the gods, or some protoreligious metaphysic guarantees the efficacy of their desires. I believe it was Bertrand Russell who warned us that metaphysical ethics is an attempt to give universal rather than merely personal importance to certain of our desires. The ethical metaphysician believes that whatever he morally desires must (in some sense) exist and can be discovered in the ultimate nature of the universe. He confuses wishful thinking with fact. He rejects evidence for a sense of self-importance, and truth for the warmth of illusion.

Justice

Consider (2), the principle that one ought never kill an innocent human being because such an act would be unjust. It raises special problems. The primary methodological difficulty is that of disambiguating the principle and determining exactly what is being asserted. The primary ethical difficulty is that of coordinating different considerations of justice; for there is justice in the sense of giving an individual his due and nothing more, and there is justice in the sense of nonarbitrary impartial treatment, namely, justice as fairness.

For example, consider the problem of euthanasia: Are we giving patients their due when, with their consent, we allow them to die? Are we giving them their due when, with their consent, we kill those who suffer from incurable disease? And in the wider sense of justice as fairness, is it fair to kill or to allow these patients to die? Few questions generate more difficulties for the advocates of the SLP, for there are few moral situations that raise more stubborn problems than the plight of a person who wants an easy and merciful death.

Perhaps the first point that strikes us when we reflect upon the problem is that (2) is not synonymous, and should not be confused, with:

> (5) One ought not kill an innocent human being because such an act would be breaking some code of law.

To say that we do not mean by "justice" merely "conformity to a code of law" is to utter an obvious truth about the language. But I think the point can be made more strongly. Not only do we not talk this way; there are good reasons why we ought not to. For once having equated justice with some code of law, consistency would demand that we call all laws just, even one that established the most vicious form of inequity or led to untold human misery. Moreover, having essentially eliminated the term "justice," we would probably want to introduce another term with an almost identical meaning in order to refer to unjust acts which are neither referred to nor covered by a code of law.

Now, one of the more popular objections to euthanasia is that:

> (6) One ought not commit an act of euthanasia because such an act would be illegal.

In normal times this is not a convincing argument. But in times when there is an almost hysterical demand for law and order, the argument gains a certain plausibility. The explanation usually given is that one is obligated to obey the law, and obedience to law is a prior and overriding moral commitment. If the issue is pressed further and one asks: "Would you feel the same obligation if you were, let us say, in Nazi Germany?" There are a variety of replies. But more often than not we are told that while there is a prior obligation to obey the law, this does not and cannot make it right to inflict or obey a harmful law. The reply, in itself, is not decisive, but it does illustrate the fact that advocates and opponents of euthanasia often agree that some rules are overriding, and that prior obligations do not make it right to inflict or obey harmful laws, generally speaking.[16]

A more serious objection to euthanasia is that:

> (7) One ought not commit an act of euthanasia because it is unjust in the sense of punishing someone when no punishment is due.

Thus we are told that a patient is usually not guilty of a crime—that he is innocent—and that to punish him by killing is unjust.[17]

For example, suppose we have a case of disseminated carcinoma metastasis before us—that is, a case of cancer where the cancerous cells have spread and have fully developed throughout the body. We know that the patient has excruciating pain; that as a result of this condition it is beyond reasonable medical doubt that the patient has to die; that the patient has earlier completed a "living will"[18] and when told of his condition voluntarily favors some means of "easy death"; and that aside from the desire to help the patient no other considerations are relevant. Now it is not easy to know all these things, and I am not suggesting that it is. What I am suggesting is that if there are such cases (and I believe there are), then in these cases it would not be unjust to kill.

Some would disagree with this analysis. The question is, why? One source of the difficulty lies in the belief that death is and always must be considered to be a punishment. This belief has various sources: the notion that immortality is a necessary condition for perfection, the belief that God punished man by expelling him from the Garden of Eden (thereby making him mortal), and the fact that human beings almost universally use death as an extreme form of punishment. Given all this it is easy to understand why people view death as punishment.

The significant question is not whether human beings have certain prejudices, as admittedly they do, but whether in the situation described the act of killing is really a punishment. The evidence indicates that the intention is not to inflict pain, restraint, or any other penalty. Moreover, the patient himself does not view it as punishment. On the contrary, he wants to die. In fact, the patient might argue that his having a "living will" places an obligation on his physician and family. Now, the question of contract is a moot one. Morally, much depends upon the nature and extent of the promises made by the family, while legally the matter is even more complex. But what is eminently clear is that in such situations the patient—if he is not actually demanding death as a matter of equity—certainly does not view it as punishment or inequity. Without contrary evidence, to dogmatically assert in the face of this that all death is punishment is like a man who, after carefully examining a black swan, refuses to call it such, because he was taught to believe that all swans are white.

I should now like to consider what is at best a moral anomaly; that is, the belief that euthanasia is merciful, but nonetheless unjust. The anomaly is the result of careless thinking, of essentially identifying the concept of being *not just* with that of being *unjust*. While the belief in its pure form is not widely held, something very much like it keeps cropping up in lay discussions.

The belief is that:

> (8) One ought not commit an act of euthanasia because, although it is merciful, merciful acts are somehow unjust.

The temptation is to reduce this "argument" to absurdity by showing that if the position is consistently held, all merciful acts—including the merciful treatment of criminals and unfortunate victims of war and oppression, and even the merciful acts of a deity—must be considered unjust. This temptation should be resisted, however, not because it is mistaken, but because such a maneuver explains little and tends to veil the underlying problems.

First of all, it is more than likely that those who hold this position have a flip-flop system of justice which classifies every act as being either just or unjust. In their universe there is no room for shading or borderline cases. Second, they also seem to hold what I should like to call the narrow view of the narrower sense of justice. They seem to believe not that one should give every man his due, but rather that one should give every man his due and *nothing more*. Third, in their opinion, merciful treatment exceeds that which is equitable, and is therefore unjust.

I think that once this view is clearly stated, it will be generally rejected. It will not be accepted that all acts are either just or unjust, since it is generally recognized that a narrow notion of equity is applicable only in those situations where such a notion is relevant as an issue. For example, given this narrow sense of justice it seems exceedingly odd to say that an act—such as the act of making a charitable donation in circumstances where it is not a matter of obligation—is either just or unjust. Clearly, in this circumstance it is only a matter of benevolence. Again, consider the phenomena of self sacrifice. Take a case in which a stranger gives his own life in an attempt to help the unfortunate victims in a burning house. Surely, without additional information that would alter our understanding of the situation, there is something bizarre in saying that the act was unjust because the victims did not deserve the treatment they received.

Nor can we accept the tacit assumption that morality is synonymous with this narrow view of equity. Even if we maintain that justice requires equal treatment in all essentially similar cases, and further hold that this broader notion of equity is somehow synonymous with morality, the claim that one ought to give everyone his due and *nothing more* cannot stand up under critical scrutiny. It cannot stand because justice is not a miser. Justice may demand impartiality in the observance or enforcement of certain rules of distribution,[19] but she does not require that we only distribute goods and services on the basis of a previous contract. She does not reduce morality to a niggardly form of obligation.

Consequentialist Arguments

The arguments I shall now consider grow out of the feeling, often an unshakeable conviction, that the SLP is necessary because its violation leads to undesirable consequences. Norman St. John-Stevas maintains that "once the principle of the sanctity-of-life is abandoned, there can be no criterion of the right to life, save that of personal taste."[20] Edward Shils makes a stronger claim, stating that "if life were not viewed and experienced as sacred, then nothing else would be sacred."[21] Although there is difference of opinion as to exactly what the violation entails, it is generally agreed that:

> (3) One ought never kill an innocent human being because such an action may (or must) lead to undesirable consequences.

Consider the most vulnerable form of this argument. Here it is claimed that:

> (9) One ought never kill an innocent human being because such an action *may* lead to undesirable consequences.

Now, many argue that (9) must be rejected. They maintain, and correctly so, that in a democracy misuse or abuse of law is almost a necessary correlate, since in a free society one cannot make laws strong enough to repress possible violations. Hence it is a serious mistake to expect perfect regulation and still cherish the values of liberty. Others say that the argument must be rejected because its underlying form is such that it can be used to oppose all political and social change on the grounds that there is always a possibility of abuse, and that (9) and similar arguments are merely clandestine defenses of the status quo; that is to say, little more than apologetics for present suffering and misery. Others go further and make a distinction between the appeal to consequences and the demand for moral perfection. The former is legitimate. A rational man must consider the consequences of his actions. But the latter, the demand for moral perfection, is unreasonable.

Aside from these pragmatic considerations, there is a logical objection that is, I believe, telling. If the only constraint is logical impossibility, then it is just as possible that an action *will not* have undesirable consequences. The result is a complete standoff. For if it is just as possible to have desirable as to have undesirable consequences, then an appeal to such consequences is completely indecisive and the argument breaks down. The argument is of little value except, perhaps, to point out that actions do have consequences.

It is interesting to note that opponents of euthanasia use a similar argument. They maintain that if euthanasia is legalized, or even held to be moral, then all sorts of disastrous consequences may follow. We reply that it is equally possible that it may not be abused. Logically speaking, the point is telling. Unfortunately, however, it is not persuasive. Following Joseph Fletcher, we then ask: "What is more irresponsible than to hide . . . behind a logical possibility that is without antecedent probability?"[22] Again, the point is telling, and again, the opponents of euthanasia are not persuaded. The question is, why not?

By way of explanation, I should like to advance two conjectures. The more obvious is that the notion of logical possibility is unclear, or is being run together with other notions. Therefore, it may be worthwhile to see if the boundaries of this notion can be more properly illuminated.

The only constraint upon logical possibility is that of logical impossibility, i.e., everything not logically impossible is logically possible. Now, the only logically impossible "things" are those events, acts, and so forth, that if expressed in language result in a contradictory sentence.[23] For example, we say that it is not logically possible for a material object to be black and not black at the same time and place, because we know that the sentence "The black object is not a black object" is contradictory. Since logical impossibility is an extremely limited kind of constraint, however, it neither marks off nor prohibits unconfirmable, false, or conjectural sentences. Hence one can say with equal impunity that the black object may transubstantiate itself into a vampire bat, or that it may not; that the man may run the mile in two minutes, or that he may not; and that euthanasia may lead to abuse, or that it may not.

The other explanation is that (9) is not as simple as it seems to be, because an important facet of the argument has been omitted. Perhaps the critics mean to say something else. Perhaps they mean to say that the practice of euthanasia may lead to abuse, and if it does, then the quality of the abuse outweighs the quality of its nonabuse, and that this is unfair. Here, I think, one has to be careful not to muddle two different problems. The first is the problem of appealing to possible consequences without any supporting evidence. The second is the problem of appealing to possible consequences with the support of evidence. To be more specific, we are now being told that:

> (10) One ought never make euthanasia permissible, because there is evidence that people who ought not die will die, and that this is unfair.

This, however, significantly differs from the claim that one ought never to make euthanasia permissible, because it may lead to undesirable consequences.

Concerning (10) and the question of fairness, I would agree that one should ask: Is it fair that people who ought not, will die because of mistakes and abuses? But fairness is a double-edged sword. One must also ask: Is it fair that those who ought to die will not be allowed to do so? Better yet: Is it fairer to prevent the many who ought to die from doing so in order to protect the few who ought not? And at what point does one draw the line? Would it be fairer to let one thousand, 10 thousand, or 100 thousand suffer in order to prevent the unjust death of, let us say, one man?

This is a difficult and heartrending question. I know of no easy answer. But it seems almost self-evident that if the criterion is to be fairness, then fairness demands that we examine and weigh both sides. Moreover, if the criterion is to be fairness, and someone must pay the piper, then the very best we can do is to minimize and equitably distribute the unfairness.

I now turn to the consequentialist argument which has the greatest intuitive appeal, namely, that:

> (11) One ought never kill an innocent human being, because such an action *must* lead to undesirable consequences.

There are many varieties of this argument, but I shall only consider what I believe to be its most compelling forms:

> (11:1) One ought never kill an innocent human being, because such an action must lead to a universal contempt for all life.

> (11:2) One must never sanction the practice of euthanasia because such an action must lead to the killing of the chronically ill, the senile, the mentally defective, the socially unproductive, and/or the ideologically unwanted.

As to (11:1): Here the forgotten hero is Albert Schweitzer, for, unlike most moralists, Schweitzer insists that the principle of reverence for life is universal in scope. Whenever possible no living thing should be killed.[24]

> To the truly ethical man, all life is sacred, including forms of life that from the human point of view may seem to be lower than ours.[25]. . . A man is truly ethical only when he obeys the compulsion to help all life which he is able to assist, and shrinks from injuring anything that lives. He does not ask how far this or that life deserves one's sympathy as being valuable, nor, beyond that, whether and to what degree it is capable of feeling. Life as such is sacred to him. He tears no leaf from a tree, plucks no flower, and takes care to crush no insect. If in summer he is working by lamplight, he prefers to keep the window shut and breathe a stuffy atmosphere than see one insect after another fall with singed wings upon his table.[26]

Schweitzer's work is seldom referred to by advocates of the SLP. At first I thought this was merely an oversight, but I suspect that there is more to it than that. If the idea of killing[27] is in itself contagious (which seems to be the shared underlying premise), then why stop at the idea of killing human beings? If it is contagious, then surely the idea of killing any living being is just as contagious, and Schweitzer's conclusion follows. But non-Schweitzerians are reluctant to draw this conclusion. Perhaps they recognize the danger. Perhaps they sense that his interpretation cannot stand, and that if Schweitzer's can't, theirs can't.

The basic issue is whether or not the idea of killing is contagious—that is, whether or not a person, group, or society exposed to actual killing or the idea of sanctioned killing universalizes and thereby extends this domain. I maintain that this question is best answered in the negative; that there is overwhelming evidence indicating that human beings compartmentalize their experience and ideas; and that it is only when the normal process of compartmentalization breaks down that one encounters difficulties.

This does not mean that human beings don't generalize. But it does mean that in the normal process of generalization there are constraints, and one of the more important constraints is that the process is limited by the concept of "same kind or same class of objects." For example, if we crush an insect and believe this to be a permissible act, we do not conclude that it is permissible to kill all living things. We conclude only that it is permissible to kill that kind of insect, or at most, all kinds of insects. Similarly, if we are taught to kill Nazis and the criteria for a Nazi and the circumstances of permissible killing are clearly spelled out, we do not kill all German nationals (although of the possible mistakes this is probably the most likely). We do not mistakenly generalize and kill all Europeans. Nor do we proceed either in fact or in mind to kill all human beings.

In other words, (11) and its cognates share a common premise, and I am urging that that premise is not true. The evidence indicates that the killing of human beings in "X" situations does not necessarily lead to the killing of human beings in non-"X" situations. Or to be more concrete, the merciful killing of patients who want to die does not necessarily lead to the killing of the unwanted or the extermination of the human species. I think this is true; but I would like to add that my beliefs are not synonymous with truth. I may be mistaken. For the question at issue is not one of beliefs, nor is it a matter of metaphysical mystagogy. It is a question of fact, and one that needs to be more fully explored by social scientists.

Questions of Ultimacy and Supremacy

Various interpretations of the sanctity-of-life principle have been examined, but thus far we have only considered those which admit or provide grounds for validation. There are other interpretations which do not possess this characteristic, and we would not be doing justice to them if we did not consider at least one other claim, namely, that:

> (4) The sentence "One ought never kill an innocent human being" expresses an ultimate moral principle.

In order to understand this claim, a fundamental distinction, often badly neglected or blurred beyond recognition, must now be drawn: When we speak of an "ultimate principle" we may, within a given theory, be referring to that characteristic whereby the principle is the final arbiter of any conflict of values. On the other hand, we may be referring to that characteristic whereby the principle in question cannot be reduced to, or justified by an appeal to, other rules or principles. In the first case, the case of "$ultimate^1$," the word is held to be partially synonymous with the word "supreme"; in the case of "$ultimate^2$," there is an overlap with the meaning of the word "primitive".

Given sentence-type (4) and the existence of this ambiquity, the following may be obtained.

> (12) The sentence "One ought never kill an innocent human being" expresses a supreme ($ultimate^1$) moral principle, a principle that is the final arbiter.

(13) The sentence "One ought never kill an innocent human being" expresses an ultimate (ultimate[2]) moral principle, a principle that cannot be reduced to, or justified by an appeal to, other rules or principles.

As to (13): It is a truism to say that ultimate principles are ultimate. Similarly, it is true, but not very enlightening, to say that if a principle in a given theory is held to be the ultimate validating principle, then it is held to be ultimate. A more interesting internal question is whether the purported principle is actually the one that is held to be ultimate. That is to say, is the notion of "not killing" the ultimate validating principle here?

By way of reply, first notice that the word "innocent" is included in this formulation. Notice also that this implies that what is ultimate is some principle of justice, and not the notion of not killing. For if the ultimate constraint is that of protecting the innocent, then it seems to follow that the ultimate validating principle is one of justice.

It may be charged that (13) is a "loaded" formulation. I agree. But I am curious to know what other formulation would be better. Is it better to delete the word "innocent" and suggest that it is never permissible to kill a human being? Or, in the linguistic mode, to maintain that:

(14) The sentence "One ought never kill a human being" is an ultimate moral principle.

Perhaps. At least it reflects the sincere belief that human life should be placed above all other considerations and that it is never right to kill a human being. To reply by saying, quite correctly, that neither the major religions nor the general literature assumes such a position, is not relevant (although it does indicate the direction in which the general sentiment lies). However, other objections, which turn on the problem of self-defense and the dubious distinction between allowing one's self to be killed by another person and directly killing (which would be inconsistent), are not so easily met. Suffice it to say that if the choice is between (13) and (14), then either one has to accept the fact that (13) is not an ultimate principle, or one must accept the consequences of (14).

As to (12): Here we turn to the heart of the matter: namely, the belief that the prohibition of killing is the supreme moral principle, and that as such it is overriding, the final arbiter. The question I wish to raise is, why the prohibition of killing and not some other principle?

There is something systematically misleading about talking about principles rather than rules. But if one insists on talking in the language of principles, if the existence of conflicting principles is a fact of moral life, and if intelligent men advance and support different principles, why should we choose this one? Why the SLP? It will not do to say that the truth of the matter is self-evident. This not only begs the question, but flies into the face of overwhelming evidence. Nor will it do to claim that all ultimate principles are supreme, for this muddles different dimensions. It is like saying that the last boy living on the block must be best, because he is last.

Instead of (12), why not say that one should always act with love? Why not say that in some situations love demands that we kill? If it be objected that a love ethic is too fulfilling, or that to act lovingly is to exceed the demands of morality, then the reply is disarmingly simple. If the love ethic is too broad (too rich, which it seems to be), and the vitalistic ethic too narrow (too poor, which it seems to be), then if one must make a choice, the love ethic is better, since it is at least rich enough to account for the wide diversity of moral experience.

However, I do not wish to give the impression that the love principle is the only one that can be successfully matched against the SLP. Indeed, I have repeatedly maintained that there are times when one ought to kill because killing is the kindest possible thing we can do.

This would follow from a love ethic, but it also follows from the rule of benevolence. The rule of benevolence says that:

> . . .We owe to all men such services as we can render by a sacrifice or effort small in comparison with the service: and hence, in proportion as the needs of other men present themselves are urgent, we recognize the duty of relieving them out of superfluity.[29]

The rule suggests that we ought to be kind; that, where we can, we ought to help those who are in need or distress.

The rule of benevolence has its share of difficulties—the problem of justification, the problem of explicating the meaning of the word "benevolence," the problem of how to determine the consequences of an action, and so forth. Nonetheless, much can be said for the other side of the ledger. Even though it is difficult to do, rationality demands that we consider the consequences of a proposed act. Admittedly, the notion of benevolence is difficult to explicate. But I think it is also true, that as compared to more obscure notions like "The Good," it is easier—note that I did not say "easy"—to reach agreement as to when people are suffering, and as to what would relieve their suffering.[30]

References

1. See: Charles J. McFadden, *Medical Ethics* (Philadelphia: F.A. Davis, 1967); Edwin F. Healy, *Medical Ethics* (Chicago: Loyola University Press, 1956); and Norman St. John-Stevas, *The Right to Life*, (New York: Holt, Rinehart and Winston, 1964). Daniel Callahan ("The Sanctity of Life" and "Responses" in *The Religious Situation 1969*, edited by D.R. Cutler; Boston: Beacon Press, 1969) does not make any direct religious appeal, but concludes that the ultimate justification for a normative principle is that it coheres with "our entire reading of the nature of things" and that it "makes sense in terms of our metaphysics" (p. 359). The interesting question is, from what metaphysic has he deduced or established his version of the SLP?

2. Albert Schweitzer, *Out of My Life and Thought* (New York: Mentor Books, 1953), especially the "Epilogue."

3. Edward Shils, "The Sanctity of Life," in *Life or Death: Ethics and Options*, edited by E. Shils *et al.* (Seattle: University of Washington Press, 1968), pp. 2-38.
4. Yale Kamisar, "Euthanasia Legislation: Some Non-Religious Objections," in *Euthanasia and the Right to Death,* edited by A.B. Downing, (New York: Humanities Press, 1970), pp. 85-133.
5. Charles J. McFadden, *op. cit.,* p. 227.
6. Norman St. John-Stevas, *op. cit.,* p. 12.
7. Albert Schweitzer, *op. cit.,* p. 184.
8. Edward Shils, *op. cit.,* p. 12.
9. *Ibid.*, pp. 18-19.
10. Margaret English, "Lead-Poisoned," *Look,* October 12, 1969, p. 114.
11. Nancy Hicks, "Lung Cancer in Men Expected to Show Sharp Rise," *New York Times,* November 4, 1969.
12. Nicholas Johnson, "Dear President Agnew. . .," *The New York Sunday Times Theatre Section,* October 11, 1970, p. 17.
13. Shils, *op. cit.,* p. 18.
14. *Ibid.*, pp. 11-12.
15. *Ibid.*, p. 2.
16. There is an added proviso to this, namely, that in cases of conflict this rule should yield to the principle of suffering—that it is always wrong to cause unnecessary suffering. Hence, in cases where this rule conflicts with the aforementioned principle, the decision-making process should be more complex than that suggested above.
17. A similar argument is used to support the claim that euthanasia is not merciful. For a reply, see Marvin Kohl, "The Word 'Mercy' and the Problem of Euthanasia," *The American Rationalist*, 9:10 (1965), pp. 5-7.
18. *A Living Will,* prepared and printed by the Euthanasia Educational Fund, 1969, reprinted 1970. "A form to be filled out by a person of sound mind and after careful consideration, indicating to his family, physician, clergyman and lawyer, his wishes in case of his own incapacity or terminal illness."
19. Henry Sidgwick, *The Methods of Ethics,* second edition (London: MacMillan, 1877), p. 263.
20. Norman St. John-Stevas, *op. cit.,* p. 17.
21. Edward Shils, *op. cit.*, pp. 14-15.
22. Joseph Fletcher, "Elective Death," in *Ethical Issues in Medicine,* edited by E.F. Torrey (Boston: Little, Brown, & Co., 1968), p. 145.
23. A contradictory sentence is a simple sentence in which the predicate term is the precise denial of the subject term. For a more adequate characterization of a fully contradictory sentence, see: Jerrold J. Katz, *The Philosophy of Language* (New York: Harper & Row, 1966), p. 198.

24. The principle of the reverence for life says that, generally speaking, one ought not kill anything, and that the principle of not-killing "must be the servant of, and subordinate itself to, compassion"; moreover, there are times when we are forced to decide which life we will sacrifice in order to preserve other lives. See: *Indian Thought and its Development* (Boston: Beacon Press, 1960), pp. 83-84; *The Teaching of Reverence for Life* (New York: Holt, Rinehart and Winston, 1965), pp. 47-49.
25. *The Teaching of Reverence for Life*, p. 47.
26. Albert Schweitzer, *The Philosophy of Civilization* (New York: MacMillan, 1960), p. 310.
27. It is not exactly clear what the relation is between having the idea and actually killing, but the literature assumes that there is a direct causal relation. Whether this is true or not is another matter, one that should be more carefully explored.
28. (12) and (13) have the added proviso, "given 'X' moral theory." For either the statements are not true, or this proviso is implied. The latter alternative recommends itself, since it is evident that the moral principle in question is not the ultimate validating principle in all, or even most, moral theories.
29. Henry Sidgwick, *op. cit.*, p. 232.
30. I am indebted to Karl Popper for a similar point.

CHAPTER 4

THE RIGHT TO DIE

EXPERIENCES OF TWO-THIRDS OF A CENTURY

Walter C. Alvarez

Soon after I started to practice medicine, back in 1906, I had to turn away a poor woman whose husband had disappeared when he heard that she was pregnant again. She was frantic to be aborted. The frail little woman had worked every day, rain or shine, as a waitress in a small dining room. Her husband was a good-for-nothing alcoholic who came home one day and made out that he was so repentant, and so loving, that she let him into her bed; the result was a pregnancy, and he disappeared. She said to me, "I already have five children; if I have another one, how am I going to take care of him? I have no mother to be a baby-sitter, and my eldest children aren't old enough to be baby-sitters." I felt so sorry for her I would gladly have performed the little operation, but, as I had a wife and children to take care of, I didn't care to go to jail.

Our cruel laws were not interested in those problems; they didn't care what a nice little waitress with no money or support was going to do with the baby. They were not concerned with the dangers of bringing up a child unsupervised most of the time, without the guidance he would need in order to keep him from mischief and from later criminal activities. What annoys me as much as anything about this bit of stupidity is that most people admit that a woman with no husband and no money has no chance to take care of a child, but at the same time they demand that she have her baby and would be glad to jail a doctor for helping her have an abortion. Women who think this way disgust me, because if they got pregnant and wanted to have an abortion and had 500 dollars, they could easily get it done. Most of them, I think would. Why can't we be more kind?

Euthanasia

In 1905, I became an intern in the huge San Francisco City and County Hospital, and for the next year and a half I took care of hundreds of old people, many of them suffering from some hopeless disease, who had come in to die. I was soon impressed with the fact that most of these people had nothing more to hope for in life. Many of them said to me, "What would there be for me if you *could* cure my cancer—or my tuberculosis? I am too old ever to get a job and I have no place to go; I have no relatives left who might possibly take me into their home, so why should I want to get well? That would only mean I would go from here to the poor-house, and I would hate that."

A few of my patients were children with their bodies or brains so botched by nature that the only thing life could bring them was suffering. I remember one such child, an idiot with part of his brain sticking out of a big hole in the back of his skull; he had another bad defect in the lower part of his spine, and as a result his legs were paralyzed and he had little chance of ever being able to control his bowel or his urinary bladder. I was glad when I heard my chief, a fine, kindly old doctor, say to the nurses and to us interns, "Don't make any effort to keep him alive." I was glad also when later the child did die, and the mental suffering of his parents was lessened.

Naturally, I became interested in euthanasia, and I have been interested in it ever since. While many people I have talked to have the idea that "euthanasia" means "mercy killing," in Greek it really means only "an easy or painless death." In my long life in medicine, I have never met any physician who wanted to take a patient's life, even if begged to do so. I have, however, heard many physicians discussing the problem often met with today, which comes up when a person with, let us say, a big stroke, has had so much of his brain damaged that he has lost consciousness and has not regained it after weeks or months. The doctors have no hope for the man's recovery; but he is fed with an intravenous or stomach tube. Meanwhile, the huge costs may have financially ruined his family. Also, the hospital bed is badly needed by patients with illnesses that can be cured.

Often every doctor on the staff of a hospital will agree it is stupid to go on struggling to keep a stroke patient half alive. But two distressing questions arise: One is, "Who is going to pull out the tubes through which the patient is getting the food and medicine that is keeping him alive?"; and the other, "When should the tubes be pulled out?" The next of kin may not be willing to accept the responsibility of giving permission; further, their lawyer may advise them not to give it. The doctors in charge may not want to give the order, and their lawyer in turn might say, "No, you had better not. The law on that is not clear." As we improve our ability to keep alive half-dead people who cannot recover, these problems of when to pull out the tubes and who should pull them keep distressing many physicians.

I imagine that some day soon a law will have to be passed saying that the question of when to pull out the tubes must be left in the hands of the patient's physician or physicians. Such a law might save the country a few billion dollars a year.

Extending A Useless And Painful Life

When I was an intern, I had an experience that caused me to do much thinking. Still today, after some 66 years, I can see the bed in my big ward in which for some six months there lay, coughing often, an old German tailor, suffering terribly from a tuberculosis which had caused ulceration in his larynx. As a result of this ulceration, every cough caused pain. I came to like the old fellow so much that one night when at last I saw he way dying, I gave him a big dose of codeine to relieve his suffering. This had such a good effect that the man slept most of the night. In the morning he was most grateful to me, but later in the day he said, "Doctor, I know you meant well when you gave me that calming medicine. You wanted to make my dying easier for me, and for that I am grateful. But now I am wishing you had let me finish my dying, because now I have to die all over again, and I dread the process." I have never forgotten that man's statement, and I think it was a good one.

A few years later, after I had begun practice as a family doctor, I came to like a fine intelligent engineer, aged 60, who was dying with a terrible cancer in his esophagus (gullet). When I first saw him, the cancer was inoperable, because it had scattered. It was eating into a number of very sensitive spots in his spine and chest, and as a result, he was suffering terribly—so terribly I could not relieve him with the amount of morpine that I dared give. Then one day, he got his very unpleasant wife out of the room and said, "Doctor, I just said goodbye to my son, who came 2,000 miles to see me; as you can see, my wife is not kind to me, so I have no reason for living any longer. Why should I go on with this dying for perhaps two or three more horrible months? Why not get my dying over with soon? You have been very kind to me, so I am asking you to get me a bottle with enough tablets of morphine in it so that one of these nights I can take a fatal dose. And with that I will be done with this agony of pain."

I promptly got the man the morphine he wanted, but that evening his wife found the bottle under his pillow and angrily threw it out. Then the man begged me so piteously for another bottleful that I went out and got it for him.

The next evening, as his wife and the nurse were eating dinner, he got out of bed and went to his bureau where he had hidden the morphine. Unfortunately, as he started to swallow the tablets, because of his great weakness he fell to the floor; the wife came running in and again confiscated the medicine.

Then she telephoned me and asked, "Did you get that medicine for my husband?" I said, "Yes. He begged me for it." She said she was going to have me arrested and jailed for attempted murder. I asked my lawyer about this, and he said, "Yes, if the district attorney wants to, I think he can make things hot for you." Fortunately, the woman did not carry out her threat.

The Right To Commit Suicide

I still think that that poor man, with his terrible pain, should have had a legal right to commit suicide, and that I should have had a right to get him the drug for which he had begged. I doubt that we doctors can help people like this, however, until our right to do so is established by law.

Because of my experiences I have read everything I could find in several libraries, trying to find out why for ages in some countries suicide has been looked upon as a sin and a crime. This was due largely to St. Augustine of Hippo, who taught that suicide was one of the greatest of crimes. A hundred years or more ago in England, if a man committed suicide, the government confiscated all of his estate. Eventually, it occurred to the lawmakers that they were severely punishing not the person who committed suicide, but whatever family he may have had, and they abrogated the old law.

Some people in Europe and America in the past thought suicide was a sin, a form of murder. Some felt it was a cowardly act; others said it deprived the local lord of a citizen. Curiously, in some countries, and in certain situations, suicide is highly condoned. In Japan, when a man "loses face" in some way, or is humiliated or disgraced, the finest thing he can do is to take a sword and disembowel himself. A prominent writer in Japan did that recently. For years, in India, when a man died and was cremated, his wife was expected to jump into the fire and die with him. That was thought the honorable thing to do. Now the law forbids it.

Sometimes, here in the United States, I have heard of a type of suicide that I thought was brave and very commendable. Thus, I can still see in my mind's eye the woman of 55 or so who came into my office years ago with an operable cancer of one breast. When I asked her if she wanted the operation, she said, "No, I will not go to such a terrible expense right now, because if I do, my son, who is beginning his senior year in college, may not be able to go on and get his degree." I greatly admired that devoted mother, and I am happy to say that when nine months later she returned, a surgeon found that the cancer, with its very low grade of malignancy, could still be removed.

Several other elderly people told me that they would like to commit suicide in order to free their grown children from the great expense of caring for them. I remember one fine mother who did commit suicide so that her daughter would be free to marry her restless fiancé.

Right now I know of a woman who is not insane enough to be put in a hospital. Instead, she will live for some months with a married sister, and as a result her brother-in-law generally must leave the house and go to his club, where he remains until the half-insane woman is transferred to the home of another sister. If this psychotic person were to ask for voluntary suicide, I would be for granting her the right, because she is mildly insane and for no useful reason she is almost ruining the lives of others.

Several able students of suicide have emphasized the fact that a high percentage of such deaths cannot be regarded as criminal or cowardly, because the person was definitely depressed or otherwise psychotic when he took his life. Incidentally, it should be noted that experts say that many deaths which look like automobile accidents are really suicides. Questioning of the family frequently reveals the fact that a man who, at high speed, drove his car into a bridge abutment had been under the care of a psychiatrist; he had been depressed, and he had talked of ending his life, which had become almost unbearable to him. Perhaps he once had had a month in a mental hospital. I feel that we physicians, and everyone, including the lawyers, should realize that so long as experts tell us that suicidal persons in most cases did what they did because they were suffering from a mild psychosis, we cannot be critical of them.

In many cases no one can ever be certain whether an apparently accidental death was a suicide or not. So long as suicide is frowned on, and so long as it invalidates life insurance policies, thousands of suicidal persons will figure out some way of making their exit from this world look like an accident.

Other Arguments And Conclusions

A while ago I was delighted and encouraged to find that that great and eminent theologian, Dr. Joseph Fletcher, Payne Professor of Ethics and Moral Theology at the Episcopal Theologic School at Cambridge, backs up those of us physicians who do not wish to keep struggling to preserve a "human vegetable." When a professor of ethics backs us up, I am sure we physicians can go ahead, as many of us want to do, letting hopeless old invalids die in peace. As Dr. Fletcher has asked, "May we morally omit to do some of the ingenious things we could do to prolong a patient's suffering . . . Unless we face up to the facts with hope and sturdiness, our hospitals and nursing homes will become mausoleums where the inmates will exist in a living death."

Recently, Dr. Maurice Visscher put in my hands a report from the *Proceedings of the Royal Society of Medicine* (October 11, 1969), telling of efforts in the British House of Lords to pass a law in favor of voluntary euthanasia. It nearly passed, but one lord blocked it by saying that it was badly drawn.

From what I read in the account, it appears that any man who now helps a dying man commit suicide can be prosecuted, perhaps at the request of an angry relative. In support of the present law against euthanasia, the argument came up that some families might otherwise put pressure on an old relative to commit suicide in order to save them from expense and annoyance. In 66 years of practice, however, I have never heard of such a case. The able Lord Platt suspected that physicians sometimes do help dying patients get out of this world more quickly and with less pain. But the point is that the people who are likely to need euthanasia are those who have been unconscious for days or weeks or years. One man I knew was kept alive but unconscious for seven years, and a wealthy woman was kept alive but unconscious for 10 years.

An interesting argument, and a valid one, was made to the effect that thousands of persons who attempt suicide and are rescued then go on living contentedly. But these people are not living unconsciously, with much of their brain destroyed. Other debaters said that an aphasic patient could not *say* that he wanted to die. And a few men raised the objection that a few people who in the late 1920's were facing death from diabetes were suddenly saved by the discovery of insulin. True; moreover, in the past two-and-a-half years, with a little oxycodone, I have been able to give back a comfortable and hence useful life to several persons who had been thrown out of work by disabling pain that their physicians had been too reluctant to treat effectively. But we cannot hope for recovery when a child is born without much of a brain or when a big stroke or tumor has destroyed so much of the brain that the patient has become a human vegetable.

Some day, of course, many people with cancer may suddenly be saved by a newly discovered treatment, but, obviously, when that day comes, we can forget the law and cure many of our patients.

Finally, I do not sympathize with the idea that if we doctors decide to quit giving artificial respiration to a man whose brain was smashed in an auto accident, we must have a court order and we must have the family and a priest present. As I must keep saying, I feel that this problem of voluntary or obviously logical euthanasia can and should be left in the hands of us physicians. Too often today the tendency is to keep up the artificial respiration and tube feeding of a brainless man. We do not have to be urged to do that.

But similarly, too many physicians, often afraid that they may run afoul of the narcotics people in Washington, are so reluctant to give pain relievers that they are letting thousands of sufferers go without relief. I think that only we doctors should decide how much pain-relieving drugs a patient needs; we must not leave that decision to the policeman on the corner.

Every so often I find an elderly person who for a few years, perhaps after a severe accident or stroke, has been so knocked out from pain that he has had to remain on a couch. By giving him enough of some pain reliever, in a

few days I might have him up and about, and soon back at his old job. I maintain that we physicians should be doing this sort of thing more often, and no politician should tell us what we must not do.

CHAPTER 5

THE EVOLUTION OF THE RIGHT-TO-HEALTH CONCEPT IN THE UNITED STATES

Carleton B. Chapman and John M. Talmadge

I. INTRODUCTION

"Medicine is at the crossroads," incoming president Milford O. Rouse warned the American Medical Association in 1967. He went on to say:

> We are faced with the concept of *health care as a right rather than a privilege*. . . . We face proposals and possibilities of increased government control . . . , emphasis on a non-profit approach to medicine, increasing coercion . . . , and emphasis on the academic and institutional environment.[1] [Italics ours.]

In striking contrast, the A.M.A.'s House of Delegates, passed a resolution two years later (17 July, 1969) that said in part:

> It is the basic *right* of every citizen to have available to him adequate health care.[2] [Italics ours.]

Dr. Rouse was stating a point of view which was clearly in keeping with policy of the A.M.A. as it was officially laid down nearly half a century ago. But the House of Delegates' action in 1969 represented a modification of official policy that may, depending on the actual meaning the Delegates assigned to the resolution, prove to be a profound one.

In linking the word *right* to the word *health,* Dr. Rouse and the House of Delegates were employing a convention that has gradually received wide acceptance in the United States. *Right to health* appears, in modified form, in the Congressional Record (Annals of Congress) as early as 1796 and reappears, largely by inference, at many points during the 19th and early 20th centuries. It came into full flower in Franklin Roosevelt's Economic Bill of Rights (1944) and has been employed by various groups, in and out of government, with increasing frequency ever since.

The meaning assigned to the phrase in 1796 was a very limited one but, even at that early date, it implied a guarantee of protection from certain health hazards to all citizens, regardless of economic or social status. In this sense, it diverged from the ancient view that health care should be provided by government—as a charity, not as a right—only to the indigent. The question of what level of government should concern itself with the right to health entered the debate from the first. And although the question, like the concept, has evolved down the years, it has not been fully resolved even in our own time.

For well over a century, the meaning of right to health had to do with health of the millions, not of individuals. In the 1870's, leaders of organized medicine specifically excluded curative medicine—treatment of the individual—from their definition of the phrase, leaving preventive medicine, as applied to whole communities and populations, to government. There was no quarrel between government and the then relatively young American Medical Association at the time.

Right to health began to assume a much more comprehensive meaning shortly after the turn of the century and the A.M.A. at first went along. But then came reaction.

Since World War One, and especially since the New Deal, the federal government has intermittently broadened its definition of right to health while the A.M.A. has clung to a conservative view of the matter. But there can be no doubt that when Roosevelt used the phrase ("the right to adequate medical care and the opportunity to achieve and enjoy good health"), he was equating it with the most fundamental social and political rights, guaranteed to every citizen. And while the American electorate has never directly expressed its view of the matter, the broadened definition has almost certainly carried the day. Very few elected officials would, at present, be so rash as to declare publicly for the definition of the 1870's. Right to health in today's usage refers to the health of the individual as well as to that of the millions; to curative as well as to preventive medicine.

Virtually by common agreement, the right-to-health question is about to become a national political issue of major proportions. Linked as it is with the recognition of a national health crisis, no federal administration, conservative or liberal, can evade the moment of truth that is at hand. Neither can the A.M.A.

II. GOVERNMENT AND HEALTH 1796 to 1846

When the United States began life as a nation, most of the states already had in force a considerable body of health legislation. Several of the original colonies had acknowledged the obligation of the community to care for the indigent sick; Rhode Island did so as early as 1662 and Connecticut in 1673.[3] Where the total population was concerned—rich or poor—the only health measures passed by the colonies had to do with quarantine. Massachusetts passed a quarantine law (against yellow fever) in 1647 and repealed it two years later when the threat had passed.[4] New York City enacted a quarantine ordinance in 1755 specifying Bedloe's Island as the quarantine site. The Carolinas and Georgia passed similar laws, also in the mid-18th century.[5]

The menace of summer epidemics of yellow fever plagued the new nation as much as it had the colonies. But the Constitution made no mention of health and Congress found no authority to act in the field of health until it was forced to do so by a crisis precipitated by a new yellow fever epidemic.

Early Federal Health Laws

On 11 September 1793 the *Gazette of the United States* reported on one of its inner pages that "Yesterday, the President of the United States left town [Philadelphia], on a visit to Mount Vernon."[6] For good reason, the *Gazette* did not tell the whole story. The President was actually fleeing a stricken city as almost his entire cabinet had done earlier. Yellow fever, which had appeared in Philadelphia in July, had paralyzed the city and a week after it reported the President's departure, the *Gazette* itself suspended publication until 11 December. The epidemic, which was at its height when Washington headed south, took 4,044 lives before it was brought to a halt by cold weather. The President attempted to keep vital government business going from Mount Vernon, but for practical purposes the new nation had no government until the epidemic had run its course. Sensing the great danger in such a hiatus, Washington wrote to the Attorney General and other cabinet members from Mount Vernon to ascertain whether or not he possessed the power to convene Congress elsewhere if epidemics threatened.[7] Since opinions on the matter differed, he asked Congress early in 1794 for the authority to call meetings outside the Capital, if "... the prevalence of contagious sickness, or the existence of other circumstances[would] ... be hazardous to the lives and health of the members. . .[8] An Act to this effect was approved on 3 April 1794.[9] On the surface, Congress appears by its action to have been concerned primarily with its own right to health rather than with that of the citizens of the new nation. But the move was a pragmatic one, initiated by an anxious chief executive and designed to keep the nation's government intact at a critical moment. Beyond this, it had no political or philosophic implications.

The severity of the epidemics of 1793 and 1794, and the paralysis they produced in the new nation's commercial life, were not soon to be forgotten. Congress might move its meetings to locations that were not threatened but the country's great seaports were fixed and the populace itself was less mobile than the Congress. Since nothing was known about the nature or mode of transmission of yellow fever except that it was introduced by ships coming from other countries, the resort was to control by quarantine. The inference of proponents of a national quarantine law was that the national government could administer quarantine action more effectively than the individual states. In the spring of 1796, a quarantine bill was introduced by Representative S. Smith of Maryland, requiring federal revenue officers to assist "in the execution of the health laws of the states . . . in such manner as may . . . appear necessary."[10] But very significantly, the proposal gave the President the power to prescribe the conditions of quarantine, a feature that stimulated lively and fundamental debate in Congress. The debate, which went on for two days, centered primarily on questions relating to state and federal authority, a singularly sensitive issue at the time. The limits and extent of federal authority in general were very much in question, and Hamilton's federalist views were strongly contested by the opponents of strong central government headed up by Jefferson.

In the House debate on the quarantine proposal, 17 representatives from 10 states took part. The principle of national, as opposed to state, quarantine was fought most strongly by representatives from Pennsylvania, New York, and Massachusetts, all of which had their own quarantine laws. Southern representatives favored the proposal on the ground that epidemics affect the whole country and "not only embarrass the commerce but injure the revenues of the United States." Representatives from Connecticut and Rhode Island (which had no quarantine laws) agreed.

Only one Representative seems to have been concerned as much with the health issue as with the question of state versus federal authority. He was William Lyman, of Massachusetts.[11] Although opposed to giving quarantine authority to the national government, Lyman, a staunch Jeffersonian and antifederalist, acknowledged that government at some level may assume an obligation to protect its citizens from epidemic disease. *"The right to the preservation of health,"* said Lyman, *"is inalienable."*[12] [Italics ours.]

This was the first mention of the right to health in Congress and the meaning inferred by Lyman was a limited one. But the question of protecting the public's health was overwhelmed by the battle over the authority of the states versus that of the Congress and the antifederalists carried the day. The quarantine measure was voted into law shorn of its provisions that were designed to give the federal government more than a permissive role in the matter of quarantine.[13] Within a few years both New York and Philadelphia, whose Representatives had opposed the first national quarantine proposal, asked Congress for a strong national quarantine law but no action was taken owing to the fact that "Congress now had a precedent to worship."[14] It was, with regard to quarantine, a precedent that would remain largely intact for nearly a century.

Three years later (1799) the Fifth Congress revised the quarantine law of 1796, strengthening the hand of federal authority to a very small degree.[15] By that time, however, all moves to strengthen the central government had come under suspicion as the federalist era neared its end. The oppressive Aliens and Sedition Laws of the previous year[16,17] had raised the specter of oligarchy and tyranny; and Thomas Jefferson (along with Madison) had, in cold fury, responded by secretly authoring the Kentucky Resolution (later adopted also by Virginia) with its extreme emphasis on States' Rights. Partly as a result, basic quarantine authority came to be even more firmly fixed in the hands of the states, a position that was subsequently upheld by Chief Justice John Marshall.

The occasion was the famous *Gibbons* v. *Ogden* decision which was precipitated when New York State awarded a steamboat monopoly on its navigable streams to Robert Fulton and Robert Livingston. The issue was one of interstate commerce but the question of quarantine authority was brought into the argument by analogy. In his decision, Marshall denied that quarantine (inspection) laws derive from the right to regulate commerce:

> That inspection laws may have a remote and considerable influence on commerce will not be denied; but that a power to regulate commerce is the source from which the right to pass them is derived, cannot be admitted. . . .They form a portion of that immense mass of legislation, which embraces everything within the territory of a State, not surrendered to the general government. . . .Inspection laws, quarantine laws, health laws of every description . . . are component parts of this mass. No direct general power over these objects is granted to Congress; and consequently they remain subject to State legislation. If the legislative power of the Union can reach them, it must be for national purposes.[18]

Although somewhat ambiguous, Marshall's opinion stood virtually unchallenged for decades. It recognized an obligation at the level of state government to protect the health of the public but made it clear that where quarantine laws "might interfere with . . . the laws of the United States made for the regulation of Commerce . . . , the Congress may control the State laws." The decision went a long way toward consolidating federal control on interstate and foreign commerce but it clearly confirmed the precedent of the 1796 quarantine law in that it assigned basic quarantine authority to the states.

But an earlier Congress had already acknowledged a degree of federal obligation in protecting the nation's health. In an action which has been surprisingly neglected by historians, Congress had, in 1813, rejected the view that health matters belong solely in the hands of the states and acknowledged some degree of obligation at the federal level to guarantee the citizen's right to health. The law was one that required the federal government to guarantee the efficacy of cowpox vaccine and to distribute it, free of charge, to anyone requesting it. Cowpox vaccination had been introduced into the United States by Benjamin Waterhouse, Professor of the Theory and Practice of Physick at Harvard, in 1800. Waterhouse sought the patronage of Thomas Jefferson by sending him a copy of his pamphlet on the subject later the same year and Jefferson responded, expressing great interest, in a letter written on Christmas Day.[19] Once Jefferson's interest was aroused, he pursued the problem of obtaining a potent and safe vaccine with characteristic thoroughness and was instrumental, in the first decade of the 19th century, in making effective vaccine available to the country's major population centers.

But the problem of obtaining an effective vaccine was (and sometimes still is) a difficult one. Partly at Jefferson's urging, the Twelfth Congress passed a law (27 February 1813) requiring the President to appoint an agent "to preserve the genuine vaccine matter, and to furnish the same [free of charge] to *any citizen* of the United States."[20] [Italics ours.] It was, in effect, a reversal of Jefferson's antifederalist stand and suggests that, where health was concerned, he was willing to modify his customary views.

The vaccination law, in principle, went a good deal further than earlier quarantine legislation and came close to demonstrating a positive across-the-board concern for the health of all American citizens up to and including the supply of the necessary biologic agent at federal expense. The law was apparently enacted with little or no opposition and remained in force for nine years. It might have remained permanently on the books had not a federal vaccine agent sent a batch of smallpox (instead of cowpox) vaccine to North Carolina with dire results. As a result, the House set up a Select Committee to inquire into the matter and the conclusion was that the 1813 law should be repealed. The Committee doubted

> that Congress can, in any instance, devise a system which will not be more liable to abuses in its operation, and less subject to a prompt and salutary control, than such as may be adopted by local authorities.[21]

Congress repealed the law of 1813 on 4 May 1822,[22] the honorable members having obviously been moved more by the outcry from North Carolina than by their concern for constitutional principles. But unlike quarantine legislation, a relatively passive exercise of police power, the 1813 act had reached out to the individual citizen by offering him guaranteed vaccine if he applied for it. In this sense, it was a precedent of considerable importance. And although the vaccination law was finally repealed on the ground that it constituted federal intrusion on the states' prerogatives, it was never actually challenged on that ground.

Subsequent decades saw a decline in federal interest in health legislation except for measures that were concerned with special groups including the military and various wards of the government. The quarantine system continued virtually unchanged except for a minor procedural alteration enacted in 1832 (for one year only).[23] The system was not, judging from the record, effective against yellow fever which continued to afflict the Nation's seaport areas, often in epidemic proportions, almost every year.[24]

But the health of the nation was, by existing standards, undoubtedly good. As its territory expanded (it doubled between 1790 and 1840), and as the center of population shifted from just east of Baltimore (in 1790) to the vicinity of Clarksburg, West Virginia (1840), food supply and distribution improved rapidly.[25] Except in a few large cities, overcrowding was no problem. Under the circumstances government, both federal and state, felt little need to consider health legislation.

III. ORGANIZED MEDICINE AND GOVERNMENT 1846 to 1910

The medical profession to this time, having no national organization, found itself at a disadvantage where health matters of national significance were concerned. The impetus for a national medical organization came from the New York State Medical Society which organized a convention of delegates from medical societies and schools primarily to discuss means of improving medical education. The convention met in New York in 1846 and laid the groundwork for the formal founding of the American Medical Association the next year in Philadelphia.[26] The founding resolution listed the Association's purposes as "cultivating and advancing medical knowledge..., elevating the standard of medical education, ..., promoting the usefulness, honour, and interests of the Medical Profession . . . [etc.]."[27, 28] Speaking at the Association's first annual meeting, held in Baltimore in 1848, its first president introduced another theme. The profession, said Nathaniel Chapman of Philadelphia, had fallen to a low state and should, through the Association, cleanse itself. But, he added, "we do not want, nor will condescend to accept of any extraneous assistance."[29] Chapman's emphasis on the profession's territorial rights struck a responsive chord; the emphasis remains to this day, although the boundaries of the profession's exclusive territory have been repeatedly redefined.

The new organization devoted its attention at first to medical ethics, education and scientific matters; but, in its first year, it urged Congress to pass a law concerning adulterated drugs and medicines.[30] Congress quickly obliged.[31] In 1849, however, the Association set up numerous committees (Hygiene and Sanitation, Vital Statistics, and others), and also sought to protect the public, within the limits of its power, from quacks and nostrums. Its concern for the public good became apparent very early through these and other actions; but it as yet lacked the strength and status to influence legislation very effectively. As late as 1901, the A.M.A. had, in the words of its president for that year (Charles Reed) "exerted relatively little influence on legislation, either state or national . . . " during its first 50 years."[32]

In the first decade of its life, the new association seems to have attracted relatively little attention in the press. *The New York Times* first mentioned it on 6 May 1858, and next day poked fun at it ("a little business and a large row") because of a ruckus at its annual meeting over the seating of a delegate.[33,34] The *Times* continued thereafter to report its meetings more or less favorably but on 9 June 1882 a *Times* editorial writer delivered a blast against the Association. The occasion was the ejection of the New York State Medical Society for not conforming to the A.M.A.'s ban on consulting with homeopaths. The A.M.A. said the *Times,* had in this action "displayed . . . an amount of bigotry and stupidity which is to the last degree discreditable to them."[35] The *Times* was also critical of the poor quality of the papers read at A.M.A.

meetings (only 20 per cent worthwhile) but, in general, press comment was either noncommittal or favorable.

The Association quite early recognized the need for a federal department of health and for federal legislation in support of adequate vital statistics. In the 70's and 80's, it was pressing at the state level for adequate licensure laws and, in the last quarter of the century, for the establishment of state boards of health. In this noble endeavor, the Association was, in effect, stressing the obligation, as well as the power, of local and state government to guarantee the implied right of all citizens to protection from public health hazards. But the policy was still thoroughly in accord with Congressman Lyman's 18th-century concept of the right to health.

A section on State Medicine and Hygiene was created in 1872 and a definition of state medicine was composed for the first time. It ran:

> State Medicine consists in the application of medical knowledge and skill to the benefit of communities, which is obviously a very different thing from their application to the benefit of individuals in private or curative medicine.[36]

A similar view was put forward in 1878 by the Association's in-coming president, Dr. T.G. Richardson of New Orleans, who told the members that public hygiene was the "prevention or arrest of all diseases which are not in their nature strictly limited to the individual . . . but which have a tendency to spread throughout . . . communities and which cannot otherwise be controlled."[37]

These semi-official definitions may be taken as the beginning of conflict between the A.M.A. and government; but at the time they were put forward, the A.M.A. was actually ahead of the national government in its attitude toward the right to health. Yet in defining public and private health as they did, the Association's leaders were drawing a very fine line, one which was even then rapidly becoming blurred.

At the state level, Massachusetts had (in 1850) taken a significant action when it set up a Sanitary Commission to inquire into conditions affecting the public's health in the Bay State. The result was a memorable report written largely by Lemuel Shattuck, a statistician.[38] In the report, Shattuck firmly points to the need for control of the public's health by "public authority and public administration." He thought the state should protect the citizen "from injury from any influences connected with his locality, his dwelling house, his occupation, or those of his associates or neighbors; or from any other social causes." His emphasis was obviously on the prevention of disease rather than on curative medicine ("measures for prevention will affect infinitely more, than remedies for the cure of disease."). But there is an unmistakable inference in his comments that the individual citizen has the *right* to be protected by government from identifiable health hazards.

Shattuck's recommendations led to the establishment of the Massachusetts Board of Health (1869) but apparently had little immediate effect on federal legislation. Congress did, however, move a year later to give the Marine Hospital Service coherent structure. To that time, the Service had been concerned solely with the health of merchant seamen and was badly organized even for that limited purpose. It now began to take shape as a health unit of more general purpose. The Act of 29 June, 1870 put the Service under the Treasury Department and authorized the appointment of a Supervising Surgeon at two thousand dollars a year.[39] Viewed at the time as a necessary but routine administrative action, it was to assume much greater significance after the turn of the century.

The National Board of Health

Eighteen seventy-eight was a major turning point in federal attitudes toward the government's obligation to protect the health of the nation and, once again, it was a massive epidemic of yellow fever that produced the change. An epidemic of the disease had been reported in Rio de Janeiro in April[40] and by midsummer had reached New Orleans. By late August the city was paralyzed and the disease had made its appearance in cities well upriver from New Orleans. Credence was given in retrospect to an earlier prediction by a black voodoo sorcerer that a plague would strike New Orleans in the summer of 1878 and that it would not begin to subside until the daily death toll equalled the degrees of the thermometer.[41] He turned out to be approximately, if not exactly, correct. By December, the epidemic had taken an estimated total of 30 thousand lives in the Mississippi Valley and, well before it had run its course, the country was in an uproar. While the disease was still localized in the New Orleans area, Congress passed an inoffensive quarantine measure requiring U.S. Consuls at foreign posts to report epidemics of contagious disease to the Marine Hospital Service on a regular basis. The new law also authorized the Service to make new rules and regulations on quarantine as appropriate provided that "such rules and regulations shall not conflict with or impair any sanitary or quarantine laws or regulations of any State or municipal authority."[43]

The action was much too weak to influence the catastrophe that was so soon to break and events during the epidemic showed with abundant clarity that local quarantine laws were inadequate in time of crisis. The epidemic ran its natural course largely uninfluenced by quarantine measures, local or federal.

The subsidence of the epidemic in November, 1878, brought with it vigorous debate concerning the best means of excluding the disease from the United States. In December, 1878, both houses of Congress set up special committees to investigate ways and means of controlling epidemics of all types of contagious disease and the

Senate's Select Committee, reporting on 7 February 1879, made a number of recommendations mostly aimed at centralization of quarantine authority; one proposal was the creation of a National Board of Health.[43]

There ensued several weeks of contest and conflict within the federal government,[44] the net effect of which was the hasty passage of a law on 3 March setting up a National Board which was charged, among other things, with "*obtaining information* upon all matters affecting the public health."[45] [Italics ours.]

The Board was organized on 2 April and included in its membership some of the most able medical men in the country; John Shaw Billings, Henry I. Bowditch, and Samuel Bemiss were among them. The Board was reluctant to accept responsibility for administering national quarantine laws until it had the benefit of epidemiologic research on yellow fever, but despite this, Congress gave it rather vaguely defined authority over quarantine in a law passed on 2 June.[46] It was hotly debated in the House.[47] Representative Jonas H. McGowan of Michigan (who had introduced the bill setting up the National Board) derived federal authority over quarantine squarely from the Commerce clause of the constitution, a view that was contested by many other members. Representative Van H. Manning of Mississippi sought to settle the conflict by resort to semantics: He noted that the word "commerce" meant much more than exchange of merchandise and must include other types of interstate and international relations as well. Most southerners, however, opposed the proposal on the grounds of states' rights and Representative Omar D. Conger of Michigan finally lost patience:

> Show me a southern States-rights democrat on this floor . . . and I will show you the man whose conscience has been relieved from all obligations as a States-rights man if he had a harbor to build within his district, or a river to deepen and improve.[48]

But the bill, which was to run for four years, passed despite the foes of centralization. The nation thus, in time of crisis, acquired its first national health authority which, although badly designed and in difficulty from the start, was the closest Congress has ever come to sanctioning a Ministry of Health. The Board was charged with redesigning and implementing the nation's quarantine system and, ostensibly, it had the legal authority to do so. But in Billings' words, "the only powers possessed by the National Board lay . . . in the character and reputation of its members and the probability that their advice would be received with respect by local organizations.[49] Its authority to initiate a research program was, however, much clearer. It was authorized to spend 500 thousand dollars as grants-in-aid for the purpose and it allocated a portion of the sum to non-federal scientists working in private laboratories.

It was, in fact, the federal government's first move to support biomedical research *pro bono publico* and, as it turned out, the Board's sponsorship of extramural research was its most successful activity.[50] It funded a large number of epidemiologic and laboratory studies, some of them quite sophisticated for the time, during the four years of its existence.[51] Among its grantees were Ira Remsen of Johns Hopkins, P.C. Chandler of Columbia, James Low of Cornell, and George Sternberg of the U.S. Army.

The Board's chief problems arose in connection with the charge to design and implement a new national quarantine system. The effort to do so quickly brought it into conflict with state health authorities (especially in Louisiana), officials of the Marine Hospital Service, and the Treasury Department. Probably its most implacable enemy was the Marine Hospital Service which saw itself being displaced by the National Board. The Board was commended for its sponsorship of research by the

National Academy of Science but by 1882 its demise was a foregone conclusion.[52] It ceased to meet in 1884 when the law that created it expired.

The National Board episode was an important but unsuccessful step toward consolidation of quarantine authority in federal hands. Probably a good deal more important was its demonstration to Congress of the value of research in the public interest. But the consensus in later years was that it was well ahead of its time and too hastily conceived to be viable.

Objections to a national quarantine authority were, however, unmistakably subsiding and an effective national quarantine law, giving appropriate authority to the Marine Hospital Service, was finally passed in 1893.[53] A Supreme Court decision handed down six years earlier had virtually invited the action. The Court at that time had said:

> But it may be conceded that whenever Congress shall undertake to provide for the commercial cities of the United States a general system of quarantine, or shall confide the execution . . . of such a system to a national board of health . . . all state laws on the subject will be abrogated, at least so far as the two are inconsistent.[54]

The turn of the century saw the passing, for the most part, of huge epidemics of infectious disease. A federal health research arm was reestablished in 1887 with the founding of the Hygienic Laboratory within the Marine Hospital Service, and funds for a building were appropriated in 1901.[55] On 14 August 1912 an act of Congress completed the conversion of the Marine Hospital Service to the U.S. Public Health Service and specified that the Service should "*study and investigate* the diseases of man and conditions influencing the propagation and spread thereof."[56] [Italics ours.] As in the case of the National Board Act of 1879, the research provision of the action taken in 1912 was clearly a pragmatic one in the minds of federal legislators: research was one means—and a politically inert one at that—by which the national government could guarantee the citizen's right to protection from disease.

Reform and Reorganization

The Age of Reform, by Hofstadter's definition,[57] ran from 1890 to 1920, his reference being primarily to reform in economic affairs. It brought federal action limiting *laissez-faire* and monopolistic practices in business, the individual income tax, and other legislation all of which had the effect of strengthening the central government. But federal action in the health field was unimpressive. There was continued agitation for a National Department of Health which came to naught despite the recommendations of several presidents and the continuing support of the A.M.A. The Pure Food and Drugs law[58] was finally passed in 1906 owing, in considerable measure, to active support by the A.M.A. The Association continued the battle when the 1906 law proved to be inadequate and was instrumental in inducing Congress to pass the Sherley Amendment in 1912.[59]

But for some time prior to the turn of the century, A.M.A. leaders had realized that the structure of the organization was too loose and clumsy to permit it to act effectively in the formation of policy. Under its old general assembly system, it was difficult to reach convincing agreement, especially on controversial matters, and concerted political action was well-nigh impossible. A few years after its founding it had disclaimed unofficial statements of A.M.A. views,[60] but it lacked an efficient mechanism for creating or proclaiming official policy. In 1901, a new system was adopted which vested policy-making authority in an all-powerful House of Delegates whose members were chosen by the governing bodies of constituent state medical societies, instead of by direct popular vote.[61] In adopting the procedure, the A.M.A. may well have been following the constitutional precedent of placing the selection of U.S. Senators in the hands of state legislatures, a practice that was abolished in 1913 when the seventeenth amendment was ratified. And by this means, the A.M.A. converted itself into a less representative but much more cohesive and politically effective organization. Under the old system, said an editorial at the time, "prolonged discussion almost always meant defeat or postponement."[61] Under the new, power could be channeled and concentrated for specific purposes. The Association retains the House of Delegates structure today. Delegates are, not unnaturally, chosen from the relatively small group of physicians, usually conservative, who have shown a sustained and active interest in medical politics.

The power structure in the A.M.A. came, in succeeding decades, to be misunderstood within and without the Association. In practice, editorials in the *Journal of the A.M.A.* and statements by its officers are usually in line with official policy but no policy is binding unless it has been approved by the House of Delegates. At times, editorials and widely publicized comments by A.M.A. officers seem to have been used as straws in the wind, like many so-called leaks within the federal government, that can be disowned if the response is unfavorable. But the one thing the Association cannot disown is an action of the House of Delegates. Even the Board of Trustees, where policy is concerned, is subordinate; it is chosen by—and responsible to—the House of Delegates.

By 1910 the Association had sought to increase its influence on health legislation by the creation of special committees, bureaus, and councils to deal with the topic. Beginning much earlier, it had undertaken to improve and standardize medical education. Probably its most effective move in this direction was the creation of a permanent Council on Medical Education (1904). The Council laid the groundwork and set the stage for a joint effort with the Carnegie Foundation, beginning in 1908. The result was the Flexner Report of 1910; but the basic work, without which the Flexner Report would have had little or no effect, was done by the A.M.A.'s Council.

IV. HEALTH INSURANCE AND THE GENESIS OF CONFLICT 1908-1932

On the national scene, economic reform and federal legislation designed to check monopolistic practices, along with demands for better conditions for the worker, were becoming daily news items. Emerging labor unions very early turned their attention to industrial safety and to compensation insurance, and in this climate, European social and health insurance schemes began to come under national scrutiny.

Except for active interest in the prevention of industrial accidents, the A.M.A. at first showed little interest in such matters. But between 1902 and 1914, 18 states passed workmen's compensation laws. In 1908, the Russell Sage Foundation financed a study of European social and health insurance systems and the resulting report, published in 1910[63] aroused the interest of a great many liberal groups in this country. The *Journal of the A.M.A.*, at the time, published no original comments on health insurance, but from 1905 on it abstracted many articles from foreign journals on the topic.

It was the passage of the National Health Insurance Act in Britain toward the end of 1911[64] that stimulated the Journal's first editorial on health insurance. The editorial said, in part:

> . . . this law marks the beginning of the end of the old system of the individual practice of medicine, and of the old relationship between patient and physician."[65]

The developments in Britain were reported sketchily in the American press but the medical profession received detailed coverage in the *Journal of the A.M.A.* beginning in early 1911.[66] The British Medical Association (B.M.A.)

had, by mid-1911, begun a campaign that was sometimes in total opposition, sometimes in favor of modifications that seemed to be designed basically to protect the physician's income and autonomy. Ultimately, the controversy split British physicians into two camps, both in effect opposed to the national health insurance bill as it had been introduced. A threat by the B.M.A. to refuse service under the new law could not, in the end, be enforced, and after obtaining certain concessions from the government, the B.M.A. reluctantly went along. The final result was damage to public confidence in the B.M.A. itself, and a legislative compromise providing inadequate coverage to wage-earners and excluding their families altogether.

In the United States, the right-to-health concept was unquestionably coming to be defined more broadly. One of the most vocal proponents of the concept was the American Section of the International Association for Labor Legislation, organized in 1906, which espoused the health insurance cause about 1910.[67] In 1911 Louis Brandeis echoed the views of the country's Progressives[68] when he told the Conference on Charities and Corrections that a comprehensive system of working-man's insurance was an "incentive to justice," and that government should not permit the existence of conditions that made large classes of citizens financially dependent. If it does, he continued, it should "assume the burden incident to its own shortcoming."[69] The next year, the same organization called for insurance against accident, sickness, old age, and unemployment. And in the same year, Teddy Roosevelt's Progressive Party pledged itself to work increasingly for a "system of social insurance [including health insurance] adapted to American use."[70]

Undoubtedly influenced by Brandeis, Woodrow Wilson lent impetus to the agitation for social legislation in his first inaugural address. Anticipating presidential health messages of the 60's, Wilson said:

> There can be no equality of opportunity if men and women and children be not shielded in their lives, in their very vitality, from the consequences of great industrial and social processes which they cannot alter, control, or singly cope with.... The first duty of law is to keep sound the society it serves. Sanitary laws, pure food laws, and laws determining conditions of labor which individuals are powerless to determine for themselves are intimate parts of the very business of justice and legal efficiency. *We have not ... studied and perfected the means safeguarding the health of the Nation, the health of its men and women and its children, as well as their rights in the struggle for existence.*[71] [Italics ours.]

Wilson seems, in all probability, to have had in mind a considerable expansion of the right-to-health concept and not to have been bound in his outlook by the rigid distinction between the public's health and private health. But his administration, so soon to be preoccupied by other matters, never followed the health issue up.

Health Insurance Viewed With Interest

The A.M.A. seems to have taken no official notice of Wilson's reference to health, but in 1914 the *Journal* published an article favorable to health insurance by Dr. James P. Warbasse of Brooklyn, a surgeon and medical sociologist. Warbasse condemned commercialization in medicine and emphasized the need for preventive health care. "The socialization of medicine is coming," Warbasse declared, "and medical practice withholds itself from the field of science as long as it continues [to be] a competitive business."[72] And less than six months later, the *Journal* carried an authoritative article on compulsory health insurance by Isaac Max Rubinow, M.D., then the nation's leading authority on the subject, urging American physicians to react constructively to the matter (as British physicians had conspicuously failed to do in 1911).[73]

Two years earlier, the American Association for Labor Legislation had set up a Committee on Social Insurance (December, 1912) which included Rubinow in its membership. Within a few months two other physicians were added to the committee, one of whom was Dr. Alexander Lambert of New York.[74]

Rubinow and Lambert were later to join forces in temporarily converting the A.M.A. to a position which, on balance, favored compulsory health insurance. Rubinow, born in Russia of Jewish parentage, had emigrated to the United States in 1893 at the age of 18. Within a remarkably short time he obtained the M.D. degree at New York University and was practicing in New York. An early interest in economics and social insurance grew to such proportions that he abandoned practice after a few years, and by 1913 he had published an authoritative book on social insurance.[75] In 1914 he received a Ph.D. degree from Columbia, and until he died in 1936, he worked actively in the fields of social insurance and health economics.

Lambert's background was in striking contrast to Rubinow's. Born in comfortable circumstances in New York, he graduated from Yale in 1884 and from the College of Physicians and Surgeons (Columbia) in 1888. A cardiologist by inclination, he was Professor of Clinical Medicine at Cornell for 33 years, and was Teddy Roosevelt's personal physician, hunting companion, and confidant. He was also very active in A.M.A. politics, serving (between 1904 and 1920) in some of its most important offices including the presidency. Lambert, a staunch Progressive politically,[76] became interested in health insurance early in his career and in late 1916 delivered an address entitled "Medical Organization Under Health Insurance" before a joint session of the American Sociologic Society, the American Association for Labor Legislation, and other liberal groups. The address left no doubt as to where he stood on the health insurance issue, and in comments on the presentation Dr. Frank Billings of Chicago unmistakably identified himself as a supporter of Lambert's views.[77] Billings, having served as President of the A.M.A. in 1903, was one of the most prominent physicians and medical academicians of the day. His reputation was unassailable, and his support was very meaningful especially within the ranks of the A.M.A. membership. But his comments got him into an embarrassing position within the A.M.A. a few years later.

In mid-1916 the Committee on Social Insurance of the Association for Labor Legislation, with Lambert and Rubinow participating, had produced a Model Health Insurance Bill, an activity to which the A.M.A. lent its counsel.[78]

In its opening sentence, the model bill rejected the term "sickness insurance" in favor of *health insurance,* "because it calls attention to the main object of the act, the conservation of health." The bill proposed that the cost of insurance be distributed on a sliding scale between employer, employee, and the state, with special provision for employees in unusually low income brackets. Benefits included medical and nursing care (in- and out-patient), medical and surgical supplies for a limited time, cash payments during illness for up to 26 weeks, maternity benefits, and burial coverage. Participation was compulsory with certain exceptions. Carriers were to be mutual associations supervised by the state. No federal involvement was proposed.[79]

The A.M.A.'s Progressive Era

To 1915, the A.M.A. had, through its *Journal,* shown only modest interest in the changing social and political climate. But in that year, Alexander Lambert, then chairman of the Association's powerful Judicial Council, addressed the House of Delegates on the subject of health insurance. His report was a detailed account of European health insurance systems, setting them out in a very favorable light; and the House was sufficiently impressed to direct, through a reference committee, that the report be brought by state medical societies to the attention of the rank and file.[80]

A few months later, the *Journal* took favorable notice of the Model Health Insurance Bill of the American Association for Labor Legislation. All American physicians should study the bill carefully, said the *Journal,* its inference being that better health insurance legislation might result if they did so.[81] Early in 1916, a *Journal* editorial, noting the introduction of the model bill into the Massachusetts and New York legislatures, said that the move "marks the inauguration of a great movement which ought to result in an improvement in the health of the industrial population and improve the conditions for medical service among the wage earners."[82]

It is difficult today to believe that such sentiments could ever have appeared in the *Journal of the A.M.A.* long noted for its ultraconservative views in support of *laissez-faire* medical care. But in late 1915 and early 1916, the *Journal* undoubtedly was reflecting the views of the A.M.A.'s leadership. To this point, however, the Association had, except for participating in construction of the model bill, taken no action. It now moved, partly at the suggestion of the Association for Labor Legislation but also at Lambert's urging, to set up its own Committee on Social Insurance. The A.M.A. Board of Trustees, which approved the Committee in February 1916, instructed it "to do everything in [its] power to secure such constructions of the proposed laws [on health insurance] as will work the most harmonious adjustment of the new sociologic relations between physicians and laymen which will necessarily result therefrom.[83] All of which leaves little doubt that the A.M.A. leadership was convinced that some form of compulsory health insurance, backed by government, was in the offing and could be made to serve a useful social purpose.

Lambert, asked to serve as chairman of the new committee, lost no time in taking action. By mid-1916 the Committee had set up offices in New York, conveniently near to those of the American Association for Labor Legislation, and had employed Rubinow as executive secretary. Rubinow energetically set to work writing, speaking, and travelling in support of health insurance. In April, 1916, he found time to testify in support of a health insurance proposal introduced into Congress by Meyer London,[84] Socialist representative from New York's east side.[85] In hearings before the House Labor Committee, Rubinow said that he was appearing at the request of the Socialist Party of America to which, he affirmed, he had belonged for twenty years. Later in the hearings he and Samuel Gompers traded verbal blows at some length. Toward the end of the exchange, Rubinow said "most emphatically that in my official position as executive secretary of the social insurance committee of the American Medical Association I am authorized to state that [the A.M.A.] is heartily in support of Mr. London's resolution, and . . . is committed to the general principle of social sickness insurance in this country."[86]

He was, in fact, too emphatic. His authorization most likely came from Lambert, and possibly from other A.M.A. leaders. But it was not a position that had been approved by the House of Delegates. London's resolution was never officially backed or opposed by the A.M.A. Its defeat, which came in 1917, was due largely to opposition from the insurance industry and from organized labor. The vote was 189 yea, 138 nay, and 106 abstentions; but it needed a two-thirds majority to pass.[87] The affirmative vote was not negligible but the defeat of the resolution was a turning point of sorts. And about this time Ernst Freund, Professor of Law at Chicago, implied that the proponents of health insurance might be pushing a bit too hard. He said that use of public funds to improve health was probably justified "upon any reasonably liberal view of constitutional power," but that compulsory contributions by employers were vulnerable to attack in the courts. "Let the advocates of health insurance agree upon a minimum program and urge the adoption of that. The well-known expansive tendency of relief legislation may be relied upon to take care of the future."[88]

In May, 1917, Lambert and Rubinow produced a massive report for the House of Delegates spelling out the details of German experience with compulsory health insurance, and describing the transition in other countries from voluntary health insurance to schemes that were partly subsidized by the state and to compulsory insurance. It also condemned "blind opposition, indignant repudiation [and] bitter denunciation of [compulsory health insurance] laws." The House of Delegates, its mood now more cautious, instructed Lambert's Committee to continue its study and to make certain stipulations concerning the protection of the profession's interest.[89]

Counterreaction From the Rank and File

But the political mood of the country, now on the verge of declaring war on Germany, was rapidly moving counter to earlier progressive trends. And within the A.M.A., Lambert and Rubinow had reckoned without the grass roots. It seemed to have gone unnoticed that the medical profession, once a remarkably unified organization, had begun to develop two important factions. On one side stood men like Billings and Lambert whose education had gone beyond the minimal requirements for the M.D. degree, who had moved from general to specialty practice, and who were prominent in academic medicine and research. It was to such men that, prior to World War I, the leadership of the A.M.A. was frequently entrusted. On the other side was the great body of general practitioners, men whose formal education was often limited, who usually had no connection with academic medicine, and whose long hours of exacting service, day in and day out, kept them relatively isolated from currents of social and professional change. The health insurance issue, combined with the rising tide of political reaction, brought them out of isolation.

Letters critical of Lambert and his committee, mostly moderate in tone, began to appear in the *Journal of the A.M.A.* and in state medical journals early in 1917. But it was Eden V. Delphey, a New York general practitioner,[90] who more than any other, converted moderate criticism to a holy war, and initiated a sharp and permanent swing to the right within organized medicine.

In March 1917, Delphey wrote that the model health insurance bill, then before the New York legislature (and endorsed by the State Medical Society), would convert physicians into mere cogs in a huge political machine. In May, he addressed a letter to the editor of the *Journal of the A.M.A.* condemning compulsory health insurance

> because it is un-American. Americanism means that the individual amounts to something; paternalism, that the individual is nonimportant but that the state is all important. Even a beneficent paternalism is harmful because it destroys individualism and discourages thrift.

He went on to say that very few Americans were without adequate medical care, and that surveys indicating the contrary were worthless because they had been done by "medically unqualified and therefore incompetent persons."[91]

As it turned out, Delphey was obviously saying what a good many of the nation's physicians wanted to hear. Many of them, in retrospect, may have read or heard Lambert's reports in silence, possibly owing to the stature of the man who had produced them. But Delphey's move opened the floodgates of opposition.

From that point on, Lambert and colleagues fought a losing battle. Lambert himself went off to war, and by the time he returned health insurance of all kinds was discredited within the A.M.A. At its annual meeting in 1919, the House of Delegates heard a final plea for adequate and informed consideration of the health insurance issue, delivered by one of Lambert's colleagues. Lambert himself, now president-elect of the Association but still in Europe, sent a strong statement attacking his opposition and urging continuing study of compulsory health insurance. But it was to no avail; the receptive spirit of 1915 and 1916 was a thing of the past, and the House now created a stalemate in Lambert's small committee by adding outspoken conservatives to it.[92]

Even this was not enough for the conservative faction of the A.M.A. Thoroughly alarmed at any prospect of health insurance and determined to close the issue once and for all, conservatives contributed a steady stream of outspoken criticism of Lambert's Committee to medical publications. Rubinow was singled out for increasingly vituperative attack. The Association for Labor Legislation, with which the A.M.A. had maintained cordial rapport a scant four years earlier, was now characterized as a Bolshevist organization in disguise, and it was claimed that Rubinow had all along been acting secretly as an agent for the Labor Legislation group.[93] On this ground, in the midst of the postwar spy scare and anti-Bolshevist hysteria, Rubinow was summarily fired, the Committee's reports discredited and suppressed, and the Committee itself allowed to die. Its last report to the House of Delegates, given by Victor Vaughan in 1920, was brief and defensive.[94] Rubinow, undaunted, continued to battle for health insurance and exerted a considerable influence on the planners of New Deal social legislation.[95]

Repudiation and Backlash

Meantime Delphey was still in full pursuit of the health insurance demon. Acting as Chairman of the New York State Medical Society's Committee on Compulsory Health Insurance, he wrote all state medical societies early in 1920, asking if they had instructed their delegates to the national House of Delegates on the health insurance issue. Subsequently he wrote all the delegates themselves, warning them against "propaganda for a scheme which could but have a serious and destructive effect upon the most altruistic profession on earth."[96]

His efforts and those of the *Journal,* which published a series of articles by the new member of Lambert's committee condemning health insurance, bore fruit. By a series of maneuvers in the House of Delegates, opponents of health insurance obtained approval of the following in May, 1920:

> *Resolved:* that the American Medical Association declares its opposition to the institution of any plan embodying the system of compulsory contributory insurance against illness, or any other plan of compulsory insurance against illness which provides for medical service to be rendered contributors or their dependents provided, controlled, or regulated by the federal government.[97]

The action, in effect, closed the door to any possibility of cooperation between organized medicine and the federal government where compulsory health insurance was concerned but made no specific mention of voluntary insurance. Involvement of local government was not specifically excluded, an omission that was soon to be set right.

The 1920 resolution against federally-sponsored health insurance was the basic dogma on which all future action in the field of health insurance was built. But the backlash within the A.M.A. had not yet run its full course. The national climate that developed after World War I was producing some extraordinary social and political results. Congress passed a sequel to the Espionage Act of

1917, permitting wholesale deportation of aliens and forbidding reentry of many already deported.[98] New York State launched an investigation on "revolutionary radicalism" which culminated in the Lusk Report of 1920, recommending Americanization through education.[99] "Within a year after the armistice," said W.J. Ghent, in *The Reds Bring Reaction,* "we were in the midst of a tide of reaction which threatened to sweep away every social achievement gained during . . . the two previous decades. By that time or a bit later the whole fabric of social control had been rent and raveled."[100]

Delphey by now had able associates in carrying forward the repudiation of compulsory health insurance and anything else that threatened to bring medical practice under any sort of regulation. Prominent among them was E. H. Ochsner, a Chicago surgeon, who directed his attacks at health insurance, health centers, and Frank Billings. In 1919 Ochsner was among the many who attacked Lambert's committee and in 1920, writing in the *Illinois Medical Journal,* he had said:

> The mental processes of some of our ultra highbrows are beyond comprehension. . . . Compulsory health insurance is but the entering wedge. If this gets by, the next will be old age pensions and the next unemployment pensions and finally . . . the last act in the tragedy of errors will be revolution, anarchy and chaos.[101]

A few months later, writing in the same journal, Ochsner disposed of health centers ("the same old baby with a new name and its feet cut off"). Quoting Billings' published comments in favor of health insurance and health centers, he turned to the personal attack:

> I wonder, gentlemen, whether we have not a right to conclude that this gentleman [Billings] is no longer a safe adviser for the American medical profession on matters of medical economics?[102]

He then went on to a number of other themes that were then new to professional debate. "When I was on the farm," he wrote, "we had occasionally to deal with skunks and rattlesnakes.... There is just one way to deal with a skunk or a rattlesnake and that is a good, dependable, reliable double-barrelled shotgun. I would no more temporize or compromise with any of the schemes so far proposed than I would . . . with a rattlesnake, a skunk, or a hyena. I would hit, shoot or kill them while they are still in embryo."

Ochsner seems to have carried his antipathy for Billings one step further. At the 74th annual meeting of the A.M.A. convened in Boston in 1921, an unsigned circular attacking Billings and quoting his earlier comments in favor of compulsory health insurance was distributed to the members of the House of Delegates. Billings was required to defend himself and he did so by recanting.

> I have declared [Billings said] in published articles that compulsory health insurance was not applicable to the United States and that I am opposed to it.

The House, apparently somewhat embarrassed by it all, accepted Billings' defense and affirmed its confidence in him.[103] It also made a weak but unsuccessful effort to discover the perpetrator of the attacks on Billings. According to Morris Fishbein, editor of the *Journal,* it was probably Ochsner.[104]

In any event, nothing quite like the incident had ever been seen in the House and, although Billings survived the attack, its chief purpose was achieved: no one was likely to bring up health insurance again, except to condemn it, before the House. Lambert, who had served as President of the A.M.A. in 1919-20, had already bowed out of the controversy; his presidential address dealt with various non-political aspects of war medicine.[105]

The Final Action: State Medicine Again

The conservative wing of the A.M.A. was now firmly in the saddle. And while the House of Delegates seems to have been unwilling to censure so eminent a person as

Billings, the language and methods used by men like Ochsner and Delphey came to be acceptable provided they were directed against compulsory health insurance. The leadership was, in fact, still preoccupied with the threat of government intervention in health. The Shepherd-Towner Act (providing funds for maternal and child health) had become law[106] despite the Association's disapproval.[107] New legislation providing hospital benefits to veterans at government expense was being discussed. As a consequence, the official policy opposing federally-backed health insurance that had been adopted in 1920 was viewed as inadequate to cover all possibilities. The question of state medicine again arose[103] and the old unofficial definition, describing State Medicine as public hygiene was, by action of 25 May 1922, superseded by the following:

> The American Medical Association hereby declares its opposition to all forms of "state medicine" because of the ultimate harm that would come to the public weal through such form of medical practice.
>
> "State Medicine" is . . . any form of medical treatment provided, conducted, controlled or subsidized by the federal or any state government, or municipality."

The definition excepted the services provided by the Army, Navy, or Public Health Service and those needed in coping with communicable disease, mental illness, and the health of indigents. It also included a loophole in the form of reference to "such other services" as may be under the control of county medical societies provided that the appropriate state society did not disapprove.[109]

The action represented a curious inversion of the unofficial definition of 1871. At that time, state medicine had to do, in the eyes of the Association, mainly with control of communicable disease and the A.M.A. approved of it. But in 1922, state medicine became medical treatment of nonindigent citizens provided by government at any level.

The official actions of 1920 and 1922, both in some sense historical accidents, were the foundation on which the organization built the image it still possesses today. The transformation of the A.M.A. from a more or less flexible professional organization to a strongly partisan one, functioning as a cross between a medieval guild and a modern labor union, was completed within a remarkably short time. The Association largely ignored a chorus of external attacks as well as words of caution from a few of its own leaders. In 1923, incoming president Ray Lyman Wilbur[110] attempted to moderate the organization's rigid new dogma in his inaugural address:

> The social relationships of medicine are so intimate and imperative that they are bound to multiply and continue. We cannot stop them by calling them Bolshevik or socialistic or pro-German but we can guide them if we get away from the brake and begin to steer.[111]

But the members were by that time in no mood to listen to leaders with the instincts of statesmen. They subsequently sought and found leaders who were not afflicted with doubts as to the wisdom of the policies of the twenties and who followed them to the letter.

V. SOCIAL SECURITY AND AFTER

Actions of the A.M.A. since the twenties have had the effect of obscuring its record during its Progressive Era, and the events that led up to it. The tenacity with which A.M.A. leaders have adhered to the policies of the twenties, despite criticism from without and within, has been remarkable indeed.

Even the Great Depression failed to shake the organization's faith in its post-war policies. Any form of interference from outside the profession—but especially from government—was to be condemned. Along these lines, W.G. Morgan, president of the A.M.A. in 1930, lectured the members on paternalism: Trade unions represented a sort of group paternalism, voluntary health insurance had its paternalistic aspects, and compulsory health insurance would allow the "paternalistic hand of the government" to throttle and degrade medical practice as it had in Germany and Britain. He also warned against nongovernmental paternalistic tendencies such as the mental hygiene movement.[112] In a similar vein was the A.M.A.'s official condemnation in 1932 of the majority report submitted by the Committee on the Costs of Medical Care, a prestigious body chaired by ex-president Wilbur and supported by eight major foundations.[113] The majority of the Committee's 48 members solidly supported the group practice concept and urged that "the costs of medical care be placed on a group payment basis, through the use of insurance, through the use of taxation, or through the use of both these methods."[114] A powerful minority, which included a number of A.M.A. conservatives, disagreed. Its report put the emphasis on "medical care furnished by the individual physician with the general practitioner in a central place," and on insurance schemes only when they can be kept under professional control. It opposed the "adoption by medicine of the technique of big business, that is, mass production." Its first recommendation, drawing its substance from the policy of 1922, urged the discontinuance of government competition in the practice of medicine except in the special instances contained in the policy.

The A.M.A. officially endorsed the minority view and a *Journal* editorial said that the majority was made up of "the forces representing the great foundations, public health officialdom, social theory—even socialism and communism—inciting to revolution."[115] The long-term effect of the decision and, of lesser importance, of the *Journal's* extravagant language is a matter of conjecture. But the decision, at the time and in retrospect, indicated clearly that A.M.A. policy-makers found their policies so binding that they could not accept the conclusions of the nation's most able authorities in the health field.[116]

Things were no different when the federal government began to look into matters of health. When Franklin Roosevelt set up the Committee on Economic Security in 1934, the A.M.A. thought that the Committee's Medical Advisory Subcommittee was not representative.[117] Even broadening the membership of the Subcommittee failed to appease the Association although it moderated its critical tone as a result. But the possibility that the federal government might bring health insurance under study was enough to persuade A.M.A. leaders that an emergency meeting of the House of Delegates was needed. The House convened in February 1935 and it found cause for alarm on several counts.[118] Most menacing was the content of the Wagner-Doughton Economic Security Bill which had been introduced on 17 January. Title IV of the bill called for a Social Insurance Board and one of its duties was to study and make recommendations as to "legislation and matters of administrative policy concerning old-age insurance ..., health insurance, and related subjects."[119]

That was bad enough. Only slightly less acceptable was the drafting of a second Model Bill by the American Association for Social Security: The proposal, made public on 5 January 1935, was a state measure and was to be introduced simultaneously into 43 state legislatures (it reached the New York Legislature on 25 January). It called for compulsory health insurance to be paid for by employers, employees, and state government. The employee's contribution varied from 1 to 3 per cent, according to the level of his income. The employer's payment went from 3½ per cent for employees making 20 dollars or less a week, to 1½ per cent for those receiving 40 dollars or more. The state was to put in 1½ per cent.[120] There was a suggestion that the federal government should put up 38 cents for each insured employee but the program was still to be administered by the individual states. To the House of Delegates, the Epstein Bill, named after the executive director of the organization that composed it, was unmitigated evil. The House of Delegates condemned it and reaffirmed its old stand against health insurance backed by government; but it yielded a little with regard to voluntary health insurance.

A.M.A. opposition to Title IV of the Economic Security Bill following the special session of the House of Delegates was, under the circumstances, sufficient to dispose of it. A redraft of the proposal, submitted by Congressman Doughton in April, changed the name and purpose of the Board: it now became the Social Security Board and had no charge relating to health insurance.[121] The new draft passed the House with 372 yeas and 33 nays on 19 April.[122] It was signed into law on 14 August, 1935.[123]

The deletion represented a victory for the A.M.A.[124] but the passage of the law led to a Supreme Court decision that politically and socially was more important than the law itself. When the law came under attack in 1937, Benjamin Cardozo, speaking for the Court in *Steward Machine Company* v. *Davis*, quoted the general welfare clause of the Constitution[125] as the basis for upholding the law.[126] In a companion decision delivered the same day (*Helvering* v. *Davis*), Cardozo, again speaking for the Court, said that the Federal Old Age Benefits provision (Title II) of the Social Security Law does not contravene the Tenth Amendment[127] and that Congress may spend money in aid of the general welfare. "Nor," said the Court, "is the concept of the general welfare static. What is critical or urgent changes with time. . . . When money is spent to promote the general welfare, the concept of welfare or the opposite is shaped by Congress, not the states.[128] The decision made no mention of health as such, but the inference with regard to it was clear: Congress might, whenever it was persuaded that the state of the country's general welfare required it, pass legislation guaranteeing the right to health and it might, also by inference, use federal tax funds for the purpose.

Meantime, the A.M.A. was moving largely by improvision as the occasion seemed to demand but always with the policies of the twenties in mind. In 1920 it had not actually condemned voluntary health insurance but its action left the impression that it might be undesirable. In a special session of the House of Delegates in 1938, the A.M.A. dealt again with voluntary insurance but said that it should be confined "to provision of hospital facilities and should not include any type of medical care." Cash indemnity insurance for such purposes was, however, accepted. Under such policies, the insurance organization pays the patient according to rates specified in the policy; the patient, in turn, pays the physician who sets his own rates. No third party should come between the patient and his physician in the view of the House. Opposition to compulsory health insurance was reaffirmed.[129]

The A.M.A.'s intransigent stands had, meantime, not gone unnoticed in some segments of the nation's press. *The New York Times* had taken a dim view of its opposition to the Shepherd-Towner Act[130] and in 1929, a writer in *Forum* said the Association's primary interest was in the financial status of the physician.[131] In the thirties, Michael Rorty, among others, pounded away at the A.M.A.'s conservatism in traditionally liberal journals. [132,133] But in 1938, even *Fortune* found the A.M.A.'s stands too strong to stomach:

> Between the elders [Trustees and Delegates], and Dr. Fishbein the A.M.A. has worked against its own purposes by clinging to ideas that rightly or wrongly have been discredited and it finds itself within hailing distance of its own downfall.[134]

By this time, few indeed remembered the Association's good work in the 19th century or its brief Progressive Era. A revolt in the ranks led by Dr. Howard Means of Boston in 1938 came to very little,[135] but in September of the same year Attorney General Thurmond Arnold served notice that the A.M.A. had gone too far.

> Organized medicine [said Arnold] should not be allowed to extend its necessary and proper control over [professional] standards... to include control over methods of payment for services involving the economic freedom and welfare for consumers and the legal rights of individual doctors.[136]

A short time later, the A.M.A. was indicted by a federal grand jury charging violation of the Sherman Anti-Trust Act. The A.M.A. and the Medical Society of the District of Columbia were subsequently convicted and nominal fines were imposed.[137] But the most significant result of the sequence was an opinion, handed down by the U.S. Court of Appeals for the District of Columbia, which held that, under the circumstances of the indictment, the medical profession was unmistakably conducting itself as a trade and not as a profession.[138] And while the message got through to some members of the profession,[139] A.M.A. leaders altered their tactics but not their policies.

VI. COMPULSORY HEALTH INSURANCE: MODERN TIMES

The introduction by Senator Robert Wagner[140] of an amendment to the social security law in February, 1939 marked the beginning of a long and bitter battle between the A.M.A. and the Senator. The amendment, called the National Health Act of 1939, was a relatively mild one and contained no provision for compulsory health insurance.[141] But the A.M.A. opposed it on the ground that it would lead ultimately to complete federal control of medicine. The bill was a principal topic at the meeting of the House of Delegates in May, 1939 and a negative report by a reference committee was, in the words of the *Journal*, "adopted . . . without a dissenting vote and even without any attempt at discussion by individual members."[142]

But when Senators Murray and Wagner, and Congressman Dingell, introduced the first of their proposals to create a system for federal compulsory health insurance and federal support of medical education in June, 1943,[143] the *Journal's* language became pugnacious and abusive. "It would," said a *Journal* editorial, "make the Surgeon General of the Public Health Service . . . a virtual Gauleiter of American medicine.[144] Subsequent editorials rhetorically inquired "does ths United States need a medical revolution? Does medical education need to be revolutionized?"[145,146] The answers were predictably negative on the grounds that the American health care system was the best in the world and that federal grants to medical schools would install bureaucratic control and destroy standards of excellence. The first Murray-Wagner-Dingell bill came to nothing but Roosevelt's State of the Union message, delivered in January 1944 affirmed "the right to adequate medical care and the opportunity to achieve and enjoy good health."[147] Over a year later, the Murray-Wagner-Dingell bill was introduced anew (24 May 1945)[148] and the *Journal of the A.M.A.* promptly took note in a hostile editorial attacking the bill and professional groups which supported it. These, said the *Journal,* were "inclined toward communism."[149] A letter from Senator Wagner, pleading for careful study of the bill and constructive suggestions from physicians[150] was published in June and a duel between the Senator and A.M.A. officials ensued. Wagner noted that the A.M.A. "has condemned every proposal which had a chance to deal with our large national needs on an adequate basis." He went on to mention specific criticisms brought by the A.M.A. and hoped that ". . .instead of pursuing a negative policy you will join with those of us who are trying to find constructive solutions to one of America's basic problems."[151]

Senator Wagner's efforts were largely wasted. Commenting at length on his letter, the Secretary of the A.M.A., Dr. Olin West, made it clear that the chief bone of contention was still the matter of compulsory health insurance. "They (the Senator and the Social Security Board) refuse to listen to any other proposals."[152] But he offered no evidence that the A.M.A. was willing to listen to proposals for any but voluntary insurance proposals under control of the profession. At best, it was a matter of the pot calling the kettle black; the polarization with regard to federal health insurance was absolute.

It was otherwise with regard to the use of federal grants-in-aid, via the states, for hospital construction. The proposal had been considered during the New Deal era and had not been opposed by the A.M.A. Toward the end of the war it was introduced as S.191 (10 January 1945) by Senators Lister Hill of Alabama and Harold H. Burton of Ohio.[153] The House of Delegates accepted the proposal in December but, at the same time, reaffirmed its opposition to compulsory health insurance.[154] The Hill-Burton Bill, somewhat amended, became law on 13 August 1946.[155]

The Murray-Wagner-Dingell proposal never actually came to a vote but was reintroduced several times. In 1945 it was first introduced as an amendment to the Social Security Act after Truman's health message to Congress.[156] The A.M.A. continued its resolute opposition throughout. The *Journal* carried verbatim accounts of various hearings and, in an editorial in 1946, outdid itself in the Delphey-Ochsner tradition. Commenting on the hearings that began in April, 1946, it referred to "the propaganda of Pepper, the diatribe of Dingell, the weasel words of Wagner, and the modulations of Murray."[157] The proposal was, in every sense, a "taking over of medicine by the state" that would abolish free choice of physicians and that would inevitably lead to "political degradation of medical practice."[158] At no time was there serious consideration of the possibility that government and the profession might come together to evolve a workable solution to a pressing national problem, something the existence of which the A.M.A. denied altogether.

The climax of the battle came in 1947 and 1948. Senator Murray (joined by Senators Pepper, Chavez, Taylor, McGrath and Humphrey) reintroduced the bill on 20 May 1947.[159] Shortly thereafter, Secretary Ewing announced his ten year plan, calling for more health manpower, 600 thousand new hospital beds, and compulsory health insurance.[160] In late 1948, the House of Delegates authorized the Board of Trustees to levy a 25-dollar assessment on all members of the A.M.A. and to employ professional public relations counsel to put down the menace of compulsory health insurance.[161] Under the direction of Whitaker and Baxter, a California firm, the campaign turned out to be one of the most expensive lobbying activities the country had ever seen. "The voluntary way is the American way" became the slogan, the threat was creeping socialism, and the American doctor could, Leone Baxter told the House of Delegates, save and preserve the American Way of Life by defeating compulsory health insurance.[162] The House of Delegates, adhering to the letter of the policies of the 20's, said that "compulsory sickness insurance . . . is a variety of socialized medicine or state medicine. . . . It is contrary to the American tradition."[163]

Committee hearings on the Murray-Wagner-Dingell proposal began for the final time on 23 May 1949, the bill having been reintroduced in January,[164] and in April.[165] But by July the *Journal* stopped publishing transcripts of hearings because "both legislators and the medical profession seem to have lost much of their interest."[166,167] For one reason or another, the battle was beginning to subside despite which the A.M.A.'s campaign continued for another two years. Not all physicians approved of the assessment or of the Whitaker-Baxter campaign; but their contract was renewed through 1951. Looking back on it all, the A.M.A.'s president (Dr. Louis Bauer) said in 1952:

> I realize that some members may have disapproved of the employment of Whitaker and Baxter and . . . have disapproved of some of [their] activities.

But without them, Dr. Bauer went on, "... we should in all probability now be operating under a government-controlled medical care plan."[168]

The Association breathed somewhat easier in late 1952 when Eisenhower won the presidency and announced his opposition to compulsory health insurance. Dingell's reintroduction of the national health insurance bill in 1953[169] caused no great alarm in the ranks of the A.M.A. But the new administration was unable to ignore the health problem altogether. In late 1954, Oveta Culp Hobby, HEW Secretary, proposed a system of spreading health insurance risks, using federal reinsurance funds, as a means of expanding the coverage of those who already had some form of health insurance.[170] It was to no avail. The A.M.A. and some portions of the insurance industry joined in opposing the proposal despite the fact that it had no compulsory feature. The *Journal* for 18 December 1954 listed 14 bills on national health program, including the reinsurance proposal, that were then pending in Congress. The A.M.A. was actively opposed to 12 of them and took no action on the other two, one of which recommended nothing more startling than a study of health and accident insurance.[171]

The A.M.A. thus made it clear that it would not willingly lend its support to any federal health proposal of consequence and that its policies of 1920 and 1922 were still very much intact. However federal planners might define right to health, the A.M.A. still doggedly pursued the view that the individual's right to curative medicine should not be guaranteed by government unless he was indigent. But a new cloud was on the horizon.

Climax: Medicare

The word *Medicare* first came into view when the Medicare Act of 7 June 1956 was passed, relating solely to the dependents of members of the Armed Forces.[172] Even so, it was thought by the *Journal* to carry with it "some danger to the private practice of medicine."[173]

By this time, the focus was on the plight of the aged and in 1957 Congressman Forand (D., Rhode Island) introduced a bill providing hospital and medical care for the aged through Scocial Security.[179] Other bills were produced and one of them (the Kerr-Mills bill), which did not employ the social security mechanism for financing, was unopposed by the A.M.A. It became law in 1960.[175] But the matter would not rest. The Kerr-Mills law required that those over 65 who were not indigent should pay 24 dollars annually for health insurance and that the whole program should be administered by the states. This was acceptable to the A.M.A.; but the King-Anderson bill, introduced in early 1961 was unacceptable because it, like the Forand bill, called for financing through the social security mechanism.[176] In any case, A.M.A. leaders considered the situation threatening enough to justify resort to a political action technique it had used once before. In December, 1961, it created the American Medical Political Action Committee (AMPAC) to "stimulate physicians and others to take a more active part in government . . . and to help . . . in organizing for more effective political action."[177] The A.M.A.'s own Board of Trustees appointed the nine members of AMPAC's Board of Directors of which Gunnar Gundersen, a former A.M.A. president, was chairman. In practice, AMPAC's chief function was to solicit funds for the support of candidates for national office who accepted the A.M.A.'s views on federal health legislation.

The fight over the King-Anderson bill reached a peak when, on 20 May 1962, President Kennedy addressed an overflow crowd, many of them elderly, at Madison Square Garden urging public support for the measure. The A.M.A. responded dramatically the next evening. At a cost estimated at 100 thousand dollars it staged its own TV show, taped in the empty auditorium shortly after Kennedy's audience had left. "This is the inside of that same arena," said an announcer, "just a few hours after yesterday's spectacle had ended. . . . The clean-up crews will arrive shortly." Then Dr. Leonard Larson, president of the A.M.A. took over and introduced the prime speaker, Dr. Edward R. Annis. The line Annis took was basically the theme of the 20's artfully framed and delivered. "England's nationalized medical program is what they have in mind for us eventually," he maintained. The King-Anderson bill was "a cruel hoax and a delusion," of limited benefits, inordinate cost, and the "forerunner of a different system of medicine for all Americans." His admonition was to go slow by defeating the bill.[178]

It was an expensive but probably effective antic. In July, the King-Anderson bill went down to defeat, although it never came, as such, to a vote.[179] But two years later a similar proposal was passed by the Senate as part of an amendment (the Gore Amendment) to the Social Security law.[180,181] The House declined to go along and efforts at resolving House and Senate differences failed.

Meantime the A.M.A. produced a proposal to which it attached the title Eldercare and which it persuaded Senator Tower of Texas to introduce.[182] It was the first time the A.M.A. had produced a countermeasure of its own design instead of reacting negatively to health bills from other sources. The Eldercare proposal was a relatively comprehensive one but still excluded the social security financing feature. The final result was the present Medicare law, passed in mid-1965, which adopted Eldercare's comprehensiveness in large measure but settled solidly on the social security method of financing.[183] Participation on the part of the elderly was, however, voluntary and in this regard the A.M.A. won a pyrrhic victory. But federally-backed health insurance was, despite decades of A.M.A. opposition, finally on the books for an important group of American citizens not all of whom are indigent.

The A.M.A.'s hope of defeating the Medicare proposal had suffered a severe blow when, in December 1964, Wilbur Mills reversed his earlier opposition to it.[184] Hope had almost been abandoned by the time of the annual meeting in June, 1965. Various explanations of the Association's failure to block the legislation were offered. Outgoing President Donovan Ward said that on the evening of 21 November 1963, after A.M.A. spokesmen had testified against the Medicare proposal, "we were on our way to the most resounding legislative victory in our history as an organization." But by early afternoon the next day, President John F. Kennedy had been assassinated and a new Chief Executive, beholden (according to Ward) to labor and liberal forces, was in office.[185] The incoming President, Dr. James Z. Appel, said that the A.M.A.'s political fortunes were on the wane because "many members of Congress—acting as political sheep—are not being responsive to the people in this issue." But he counselled against boycott, if the law should pass;[186] and in this he was subsequently supported by the Board of Trustees.[187]

The passage of Medicare and other health legislation thus left the Association's leaders disgruntled and bewildered but not openly rebellious. And in 1968, another incoming president inquired in his inaugural address:

> Will we learn the lessons of our experience, particularly those that led to the laws affecting health that were passed by the 89th Congress?

He followed his question by a plea for enlightened guidance by the Association of the federal health planning process; steering rather than braking.[188] It was basically the same plea that had been made, and ignored, 45 years earlier by Ray Lyman Wilbur; and it was his son, Dwight L. Wilbur, who eloquently restated it in 1968.

VII. SUMMARY AND PROSPECTS FOR THE 70'S

Neither the federal government nor the A.M.A. is irreversibly committed to its precedents; nor is either likely to be uninfluenced by them. Since the first quarantine law was enacted in 1796, the federal definition of the right to health has been steadily broadened. But except for the short-lived vaccination law of 1813, federal health legislation did not begin to approach a guarantee of adequate health services to individual American citizens until comparatively modern times. With the passage of the Social Security Law in 1935, and the Cardozo decision two years later, a new climate was created. The several health bills introduced by Senator Robert Wagner and colleagues beginning in 1939 followed in due course. The passage of the Medicare-Medicaid Law and other health legislation in 1965 brought the process to its present state.

Since its founding in 1848, the A.M.A. has played a key role in the development and passage of health legislation. Prior to the passage of Social Security, the federal government and the A.M.A., for the most part, saw comfortably eye-to-eye. As long as the definition of the right to health was a conservative one—encompassing the health of the millions but not curative medicine for the individual—the A.M.A. was, in fact, ahead of government, federal and state. The Model Health Insurance Bill of 1916, which the A.M.A. helped to draft, was the real beginning of conflict. It embodied compulsory health insurance, financed by tripartite contributions: employee, employer and state (but not federal) government. The Association's policies of 1920 and 1922 declared the proposal, and most others in which government control and financing are involved, to be anathema. The stage was then set for the battles over Social Security, the various Wagner bills, and those having to do with health care for the elderly. In the course of the long struggle, the A.M.A. has ceded very little. The Kerr-Mills Law, which the Association approved, focussed on the states, held the federal government more or less at arm's length, and did no great violence to the A.M.A.'s view that only the indigent should receive personal health services at taxpayer's expense. But the Forand Bill and its successors put the federal government in the central position and extended benefits to all eligibles, regardless of economic status. In this sense Medicare was a watershed; it breached the A.M.A.'s 1922 definition of state medicine solidly and definitely. The extension of the Medicare system to virtually all citizens (and the revision or elimination of the state-oriented Medicaid provision), or possibly a new law having the same effect, is the prospect of the 70's.

Few organizations in American history have been so thoroughly dissected and criticized as the A.M.A. Some of the analyses [189 - 192] are scholarly and relatively dispassionate; others are strident and doctrinaire. Many have predicted that unless the A.M.A. changes its ways, it is headed for oblivion. But the Association has ignored them all and has doggedly gone its conservative way. It is a remarkably durable institution; dire prophecies of oblivion, some dating back many decades, show little sign of becoming fact. But the Association's tactics have changed remarkably. Gone are the editorial polemics against the federal government in the *Journal*, and so are full extracts of the Minutes of the House of Delegates. The Association's *American Medical News* and *Today's Health* both reflect its political and social point of view.

but reports are likely to be more reportorial and less overtly propagandistic than formerly. Nor is there any suggestion that the spectacular Madison Square Garden countermeasure of 1962 will be repeated in the foreseeable future. Yet the Delphey-Ochsner style has not completely disappeared. It cropped up recently in a letter to the editor of the *American Medical News* when an A.M.A. constituent described the *News* as a "blatant organ of the left-wing conspiracy."[193]

It is hardly that. But in the face of mounting pressure for national health insurance, the A.M.A. has put forward its own plan to which it applies the title Medicredit.[194,195] The proposal is based on a scale of federal income tax credit to encourage the voluntary purchase of health insurance from existing organizations, private and semi-public. It would not alter the existing fee-for-service system nor does it contain specific inducements for physicians to locate in low-income or rural areas. It is basically a voluntary financing measure, not one that is designed to create a new health care system. At the opposite pole is a proposal backed by the Committee for National Health Insurance. It calls for compulsory health insurance for everyone and embodies the tripartite (employer, employee, and government) financing system put forward by the Model Bill of 1916.[196] It would virtually abolish fee-for-service practice and private health insurance plans. It would provide "financial and other" incentives to physicians willing to form medical care groups and to those who move into various low-income areas. It would assign highest priority in payment of funds collected by the system to salaried physicians in institutions, to those working in group practice prepayment units, and to physicians who agree to "accept capitation payments for the care of a defined population."[197]

It is difficult to see how more features that have traditionally been repugnant to the A.M.A. could be incorporated into a single health insurance proposal. The Association's strenuous opposition to some features of the Committee's proposal is a certainty. It is not likely, however, to go back to the tactics of the 40's, 50's and early 60's. For one thing, the Association's approach to the public is more sophisticated than it was then. For another, the A.M.A.'s political arm (AMPAC) is said to exert more direct influence on the White House than was the case in earlier administrations.[198] But nothing that took place at the 1970 A.M.A. Convention suggests that the A.M.A. is as yet ready to reconsider all the present implications of its policies of the 20's.[199]

The dilemma the A.M.A. faces in the early 70's is, in many respects, more stringent than that faced by the present Administration in Washington. The latter is as yet committed to nothing, beyond the recognition by the President of a health crisis. It can move in many directions, according to its sense of public opinion and the mood of Congress. But the A.M.A. still labors under the self-imposed strictures of the 20's and the disadvantages under which it must now work are formidable. It must, on the one hand, continue to represent the interests of its members; and it must, on the other hand, participate in the creation of a system that will finally guarantee the right to health of all American citizens. The Association is not wrong in pointing out the dangers inherent in a health care system that is controlled absolutely by government; it could as well point out the obvious dangers of complete control by the consumer. But it cannot continue to confuse professional control of health care standards with professional control of the system itself.

To play its vital role in the guarantee of the right to health in the 70's, the A.M.A. needs to reconsider its own precedents. Those of 1920 and 1922, developed in time of great political stress, stand today in sharp contrast to the enlightened and relevant precedents of earlier times. The policies of the 20's, more than anything else, have brought the Association to its present dilemma.

Its future may well depend on how convincingly it can rewrite—or expunge—those policies and on whether or not the House of Delegates' resolution of 1969 really means what it seems to say:

> It is the basic right of every citizen to have available to him adequate health care.

References

1. Rouse, Milford O.: Inaugural Address: To Whom Much Has Been Given. JAMA 201:169-171, 17 July 1967.
2. A.M.A. Convention news. New York Times. 18 July 1969, p. 21.
3. Capen, Edward Warren: The Historical Development of the Poor Law of Connecticut. New York; Columbia University Press, 1905.
4. Records of the Governor and Company of the Massachusetts Bay in New England, 1642-1649 2:237, March 1647-8. Boston: William White, 1853.
5. Gordon, Maurice Bear: Aesculapius Comes to the Colonies. Ventnor N.J.: Ventnor Publishers, Inc., 1949.
6. Gazette of the United States. 11 September 1793, p. 535.
7. Washington, George: Letter to the Attorney General; Mt. Vernon, 30 September 1793. In: Writings of Washington 33:107-109. Washington: U.S. Govt. Printing Office, 1940.
8. Gazette of the United States. 2 April 1794, p. 2-3.
9. An Act to Authorize the President of the United States in Certain Cases to Alter the Place for Holding a Session of Congress. Third Cong., 1st Sess. Pub. Stat. at Large U.S. 1:353, 3 April 1794.
10. Gazette of the United States. 29 April 1796, p. 2.
11. Lyman, born at Northampton in 1755, served in the House from 1793 to 1797. He belonged to the most radical wing of ths Jeffersonian Party and was later rewarded by Jefferson with a Consulship in London. He died in England in 1811 and is interred at Gloucester Cathedral. (Dexter, Franklin B.: Biographical Sketches of the Graduates of Yale College 3:619-620, 1903. New York: H. Holt and Company, 1885-1913.)
12. Lyman, William: Comment in House of Representatives. Fourth Cong., 1st Sess. Cong. Rec. (Ann. Cong.), 11 May 1796, p. 1348.
13. An Act Relative to Quarantine. Fourth Cong., 1st Sess. Pub. Stat. at Large U.S. 1:474, 27 May 1796.
14. Allen, William H.: The Rise of the National Board of Health. Ann. Amer. Acad. Polit. and Soc. Sci. 15:51-68, January-May, 1900.

15. An Act Respecting Quarantine and Health Laws. Fifth Cong., 3rd Sess. Pub. Stat. at Large U.S. 1:619, 25 February 1799.
16. An Act Concerning Aliens. Fifth Cong., 2nd Sess. Pub. Stat. at Large U.S. 1:570-572, 25 June 1798.
17. An Act in Addition to the Act, Entitled "An Act for the Punishment of Certain Crimes Against the United States." Fifth Cong., 2nd Sess. Pub. Stat. at Large U.S. 1:596-597, 14 July 1798.
18. Gibbons *vs.* Ogden. Reports of Cases Argued and Adjudged by the Supreme Court of the United States (Wheaton); February term 9:1-222, 1824, p. 203.
19. Martin, Henry A.: Jefferson as a Vaccinator. North Carolina Med. J. 7:1-34, January, 1881.
20. An Act to Encourage Vaccination. Twelfth Cong., 2nd Sess. Pub. Stat. at Large U.S. 2:806-807, 27 February 1813.
21. Report of the Select Committee . . . to Inquire Into the Propriety of Repealing the Act of 1813, to Encourage Vaccination, Accompanied With a Bill to Repeal the Act, Entitled "An Act to Encourage Vaccination." Seventeenth Cong., 1st Sess. House Report No. 93, 13 April 1822.
22. An Act to Repeal the Act Entitled "An Act to Encourage Vaccination." Seventeenth Cong., 1st Sess. Pub. Stat. at Large U.S. 3:677, 4 May 1822.
23. An Act to Enforce Quarantine Regulations. Twenty-second Cong., 1st Sess. Pub. Stat. at Large U.S. 4:577-578, 13 July 1832.
24. Keating, J.M.: A History of the Yellow Fever. The Yellow Fever Epidemic of 1878 in Memphis, Tenn. Memphis: The Howard Association, 1879, p. 327-443.
25. The 1970 World Almanac and Book of Facts. New York: Newspaper Enterprise Asso., Inc., 1969, p. 254.
26. Evening Post (New York). 6 May 1846, p. 2.
27. Proceedings of ths National Medical Conventions Held in New York, May, 1846, and in Philadelphia, May, 1847. Philadelphia: T.K. and P.G. Collins, Printers, 1847.
28. Davis, N.S.: History of the American Medical Association From Its Organization up to January, 1855. Philadelphia: Lippincott, Grambo, and Co., 1855.
29. Chapman, Nathaniel: President's Address. Trans. Amer. Med. Asso. 1:7-9, 1848.
30. Memorial to Congress on Adulterated Drugs and Medicines. Trans. Amer. Asso. Med. 1:335, 4 May 1848.
31. An Act to Prevent the Importation of Adulterated and Spurious Drugs and Medicine. Thirtieth Cong., 1st Sess. Pub. Stat. at Large U.S. 9:237-239, 26 June 1848.

32. Reed, Charles: President's Address. JAMA 36:1599-1606, 8 June 1901.
33. Editorial: The Medical Association. New York Times, 6 May 1858, p. 1.
34. Editorial: American Medical Association. A Little Business and a Large Row. New York Times, 7 May 1858, p. 1.
35. Editorial: Medical Ethics. New York Times, 9 June 1882, p. 4.
36. Logan, Thomas M.: Report of the Committee on a National Health Council. Trans. Amer. Med. Asso. 23:46-51, 9 May 1872.
37. Richardson, T.G.: Presidential Address. Twenty-Ninth Annual Meeting. Trans. Amer. Med. Asso. 29:93-111, 1878, p. 111.
38. Commissioners of the Sanitary Survey: Report of a General Plan for the Promotion of Public and Personal Health ... [Lemuel Shattuck]. Boston: Dutton and Wentworth, 1850, p. 10.
39. An Act to Reorganize the Marine Hospital Service and to Provide for the Relief of Sick and Disabled Seamen. Forty-first Cong., 2nd Sess. Pub. Stat. at Large U.S. 16:169-170. 29 June 1870.
40. Yellow Fever at Rio de Janeiro. New York Times, 17 April 1878, p. 8.
41. Desolation in the South. New York Times, 5 September 1878, p. 1.
42. An Act to Prevent the Introduction of Contagious or Infectious Diseases Into the United States. Forty-fifth Cong., 2nd Sess. Pub. Stat. at Large U.S. 20:37-38, 29 April 1878.
43. Senate Report No. 734; to Accompany S.1784. Forty-fifth Cong., 3rd Sess. 7 February 1879.
44. Cabell, J.L.: A Review of the Operations of the National Board of Health. Rep. Amer. Pub. Health Asso. 8:71-101, 1883.
45. An Act to Prevent the Introduction of Infectious or Contagious Diseases Into the United States, and to Establish a National Board of Health. Forty-fifth Cong., 3rd Sess. Pub. Stat. at Large U.S. 20:484-485, 3 March 1879.
46. An Act to Prevent the Introduction of Contagious or Infectious Diseases Into the United States. Forty-sixth Cong., 1st Sess. Pub. Stat. at Large U.S. 21:5-7, 2 June 1879.
47. Debate on Quarantine Act of 2 June 1879. Forty-sixth Cong., 1st Sess. Cong. Rec. 9(2):1637-1650, 27 May 1879.
48. *Ibid.*
49. Billings, John Shaw: Reports and Resolutions Relating to Sanitary Legislation. Amer. J. Med. Sci. 78:471-479, October, 1879.
50. The practice of awarding research grants to private individuals working in non-federal institutions was reinstated briefly during World War I. In 1937 it was incorporated in the National Cancer Act and, from 1948 onward, formed a major feature of the vastly expanded activities of the National Institutes of Health.
51. Cabell, J.L., *op. cit.* (note 44).

52. Editorial: The National Board of Health and the American Public Health Association. Boston Med. and Surg. J. 107:450-451, 9 November 1882.
53. An Act Granting Additional Quarantine Powers and Imposing Additional Duties Upon the Marine-Hospital Service. Fifty-second Cong., 2nd Sess. Pub. Stat. at Large U.S. 27:449-452, 15 February 1893.
54. Morgan's Louisiana and Texas Railroad and Steamship Company *vs.* Board of Health of the State of Louisiana and the State of Louisiana. U.S. Supreme Court Reps. (Lawyers Edition) 30:237-243, 10 May 1886.
55. An Act Making Appropriations for Sundry Civil Expenses of the Government for the Fiscal Year Ending June Thirtieth, 1902, and for Other Purposes. Fifty-sixth Cong., 2nd Sess. Pub. Stat. at Large U.S. 31:1137, 3 March 1901.
56. An Act to Change the Name of the Public Health and Marine Hospital Service to the Public Health Service, to Increase the Pay of Officers of Said Service, and for Other Purposes. Sixty-second Cong., 2nd Sess. Pub. Stat. at Large U.S. 37(1):309, 14 August 1912.
57. Hofstadter, Richard: The Age of Reform; From Bryan to F.D.R. New York: Alfred Knopf, 1955, 328 p.
58. An Act for Preventing the Manufacture, Sale, or Transportation of Adulterated or Misbranded or Poisonous or Deleterious Food, Drugs, Medicines, and Liquors, and for Regulating Traffic Therein, and for Other Purposes. Fifty-ninth Cong., 1st Sess. Pub. Stat. at Large U.S. 34(1):768-772, 30 June 1906.
59. An Act to Amend Section Eight of the Food and Drugs Act Approved June Thirtieth, Nineteen Hundred and Six. Sixty-second Cong., 2nd Sess. Pub. Stat. at Large U.S. 37(1):416-417, 23 August 1912.
60. Resolution on Official Policy of the Association. Trans. Amer. Med. Asso. 4:39, 9 May 1851.
61. Official Minutes of the General Sessions: Report of the Transactions of the Reorganization Committee on Revision of Constitution and By-laws. JAMA 36:1643-1648, 8 June 1901.
62. Editorial: The House of Delegates. American Medicine 3:1030, 21 June 1902.
63. Frankel, Lee K., and Dawson, Miles M.: Workman's Insurance in Europe, New York: Charities Publication Committee, 1910.
64. It went into force on 1 July 1912.
65. Editorial: Socializing the British Medical Profession. JAMA 59:1890-1891, 23 November 1912.
66. In the form of *London Letters,* written by a correspondent. The first to deal with the British health insurance proposal appeared on 3 June 1911. There were about 30 of them over the next eighteen months.
67. The American Association held its first meeting in Madison, Wisconsin 30-31 December 1907 and was disbanded in 1942.

68. Members of a political movement which was later to become Theodore Roosevelt's "Bull Moose" third party.
69. Brandeis, Louis D.: Workingman's Insurance—The Road to Social Efficiency. Proc. Conf. of Charities and Corrections, 38th Annual Session, 8 June 1911, p. 156-162.
70. A Contract With the People. Platform of the Progressive Party Adopted at Its First National Convention. Chicago, 7 August 1912. New York: Progressive National Committee, 1912.
71. Wilson, Woodrow: First Inaugural Address as President of the United States, 4 March 1913. The Public Papers of Woodrow Wilson. The New Democracy, vol. 1. New York: Harper and Brothers, 1926.
72. Warbasse, James P.: The Socialization of Medicine. JAMA 63:264-266, 18 July 1914.
73. Rubinow, Isaac M.: Social Insurance and the Medical Profession. JAMA 64:381-386, 30 January 1915.
74. American Association for Labor Legislation. Annual Business Meeting, December 1912. Amer. Labor Legislation Rev. 3:121, 1913.
75. Rubinow, I.M.: Social Insurance, With Special Reference to American Conditions. New York: Henry Holt and Company, 1913.
76. The leadership of the Progressive Party, as studied by Chandler, was upper middle class. Most had earlier been Republicans and most were businessmen, lawyers, editors, or university professors, in that order. Very few were physicians. (Chandler, Alfred D.: The Origins of Progressive Leadership. In: The Letters of Theodore Roosevelt. Vol. 8, Elting Morrison, ed. Cambridge: Harvard University Press, 1954, pp. 1462-1465.)
77. Lambert, Alexander: Medical Organization Under Health Insurance. Amer. Labor Legislation Rev. 7:36-50, March, 1917.
78. Editorial: Industrial Insurance. JAMA 66:433, 5 February 1916.
79. Health Insurance: Tentative Draft of an Act. Amer. Labor Legislation Rev. 6:239-268, June 1916. The signal importance of the model bill seems to have been largely forgotten in our own time. Drafted with great care, it avoided some of the defects of European systems and has influenced planners, directly or indirectly, ever since. Neither federal nor state government was involved in its preparation. It was introduced into the New York legislature with Governor Al Smith's endorsement; it passed the Senate but was defeated in the House. Commissions to study the proposal were set up in California, Illinois, New Jersey, Ohio, Pennsylvania, Wisconsin and others. Some reports were favorable but no legislation resulted.
80. Minutes of House of Delegates: Report of the Judicial Council of the House of Delegates [21 June]. JAMA 65:73-92, 3 July 1915.
81. Current Comment: A Model Bill for Health Insurance. JAMA 65:1824, 20 November 1915.

82. Editorial: Cooperation in Social Insurance Investigation. JAMA 66:1469-1470, 6 May 1916.
83. Minutes of House of Delegates: Report of Committee on Social Insurance. JAMA 66:1951-1985, 17 June 1916.
84. London, like Rubinow, was born in Russia (1871). He came to the United States in 1891 and served in the 64th, 65th and 66th Congresses representing the 12th New York District. Also like Rubinow, he was an active supporter of the American Association for Labor Legislation. (Rogoff, Hillel: An East Side Epic; the Life and Work of Meyer London. New York: Vanguard Press, 1930.)
85. House Joint Resolution 159: For the Appointment of a Commission to Prepare and Recommend a Plan for the Establishment of a National Insurance Fund, and for the Mitigation of the Evil of Unemployment. Sixty-fourth Cong., 1st Sess. Cong. Rec. 53:2856, 19 February 1916.
86. Hearings Before the Committee on Labor (HR): Commission to Study Social Insurance and Unemployment. April 6 and 11, 1916. Sixty-fourth Cong., 1st Sess. Washington: U.S. Govt. Printing Office, 1916.
87. Debate on National Insurance. Sixty-fourth Cong., 2nd Sess. Cong. Rec. 54(3):2650-2654, 5 February 1917.
88. Freund, Ernst: Constitutional and Legal Aspects of Health Insurance. Nat. Conf. Social Work 1917:553-558.
89. Minutes of House of Delegates: Reports of Committee on Social Insurance Regarding Invalidity, Old Age, and Unemployment Insurance, and a General Summary Concerning Social Insurance. JAMA 68:1721-1755, 9 June 1917.
90. Eden Vinson Delphey (1858-1925) graduated from the Medical Department of Columbia College in 1889 and practiced at 171 W. 71st Street for many years.
91. Delphey, Eden V.: Arguments Against the "Standard Bill" for Compulsory Health Insurance. JAMA 68:1500-1501, 19 May 1917.
92. Minutes of House of Delegates: Report of the Council on Health and Public Instruction. JAMA 72:1750-1751, 14 June 1919.
93. Fishbein, Morris: History of the American Medical Association. Philadelphia: W.B. Saunders Company, 1947, p. 318.
94. Minutes of House of Delegates: Report of Committee on Social Insurance. JAMA 74:1241-1242, 1 May 1920.
95. Rubinow, chairing a session on health insurance at the Seventh National Conference on Social Security in 1934 said:

" . . . I feel that I am called upon to give a word of caution, which may partly be explained by my own age. I don't look forward to waiting another thirty or forty years before these various research programs... culminate in a system. I can't help feeling a little bit depressed... by the fact that so much that has been said here this morning has been said... some twenty years ago. . . ."

(Wanted—A Health Insurance Program. In: Social Security in the United States, 1934, p. 12. New York: American Association for Social Security, 1934.)

Rubinow died in September, 1936.

96. Delphey, Eden V.: Report of the Committee on Compulsory Health and Workmen's Compensation Insurance of the Medical Society of the County of New York. New York State J. Med. 20:394-396, December, 1920.
97. Minutes of House of Delegates: Report of Reference Committee on Hygiene and Public Health (27 April). JAMA 74:1319, 8 May 1920.
98. An Act to Deport Certain Undesirable Aliens and to Deny Readmission to Those Deported. Sixty-sixth Cong., 2nd Sess. Pub. Stat. at Large U.S. 41(1):593-594, 10 May 1920.
99. Lusk, Clayton R. (Chairman): Revolutionary Radicalism. . . . Report of the Joint Legislative Committee [Lusk Report], 4 vols. Albany: J.B. Lyon Co., 1920.
100. Ghent, W.J.: The Reds Bring Reaction. Princeton: Princeton University Press, 1923.
101. Ochsner, Edward H.: Compulsory Health Insurance, a Modern Fallacy. Illinois Med. J. 38:77-80, August, 1920.
102. Ochsner, Edward H.: Some Medical Economics Problems. Illinois Med. J. 39:406-413, May, 1921.
103. Minutes of House of Delegates for 9 June 1921. JAMA 76:1757-1758, 18 June 1921.
104. Fishbein, Morris: History of the American Medical Association. Philadelphia: W.B. Saunders Company, 1947, p. 324-325.
105. Lambert, Alexander: Medicine, a Determining Factor in War. Presidential Address. JAMA 72:1713-1721, 14 June 1919.
106. An Act for the Promotion of the Welfare and Hygiene of Maternity and Infancy, and for Other Purposes (P.L.67-97). Sixty-seventh Cong., 1st Sess. Pub. Stat. at Large U.S. 42(1):224-226, 23 November 1921.
107. Editorial: Federal Care of Maternity and Infancy. The Shepherd-Towner Bill. JAMA 76:383, 5 February 1921.
108. It had come up at the 1921 annual session. Delphey had introduced a resolution defining state medicine as "... the practice of medicine by the state by physicians on a salary to the exclusion of all other and individual practice of medicine." His resolution, and several other similar ones, were buried in various committees. (Minutes of House of Delegates: Various Resolutions. JAMA 76:1756-1757, 18 June 1921.)
109. Minutes of House of Delegates 25 May 1922. Supplementary Report of Reference Committee on Legislation and Public Relations. JAMA 78:1715, 3 June 1922.
110. Ray Lyman Wilbur (1875-1949) was one of the most distinguished men of his time. He was an accomplished physician, President of

Stanford from 1916 to 1943, Secretary of the Interior in Hoover's cabinet (1929-1933), President of the AMA in 1923-24 and President of the Association of American Medical Colleges in 1924.
111. Wilbur, Ray Lyman: Human Welfare and Modern Medicine. Inaugural Address. JAMA 80:1889-1893, 30 June 1923.
112. Morgan, William G.: The Medical Profession and the Paternalistic Tendencies of the Times. President's Address. JAMA 94:2035-2042, 28 June 1930.
113. The Carnegie Corporation, the Josiah Macy, Jr. Foundation, the Milbank Memorial Fund, the New York Foundation, the Rockefeller Foundation, the Julius Rosenwald Fund, the Russell Sage Foundation, and the Twentieth Century Fund.
114. Committee on the Costs of Medical Care: Medical Care for the American People: The Final Report. Chicago: University of Chicago Press, 1932 (Publication No. 28).
115. Editorial: The Committee on the Costs of Medical Care. JAMA 99:1950-1952, 3 December 1932.
116. The Committee (17 practicing physicians and dentists, six public health authorities, six social scientists, ten representatives of health institutions, and nine members representing the public) could hardly have been more carefully chosen. Eight of the 15 practicing physicians, and one Ph.D., wrote the minority report. The two dentists also submitted a minority report. One social scientist submitted a critical personal statement and Edgar Sydenstricker (public health) declined to sign the final report because, in his view, it dealt inadequately with "the fundamental economic question which the Committee was formed... to consider." The majority report was supported by 35 of the 48 members.
117. Editorial: The Conference on Economic Security. JAMA 103:1624-1625, 24 November 1934.
118. Minutes of ths Special Session of the House of Delegates of the American Medical Association, Chicago, 15-16 February 1935. JAMA 104:747-753, 2 March 1935.
119. The Economic Security Act (S.1130). Seventy-fourth Cong., 1st Sess. Cong. Rec. 79(1):549-556, 17 January 1935.
120. Model Bill Maps Health Insurance. New York Times, 6 January 1935, Sec. 2, p. 2.
121. A Bill (H.R. 7260) to Provide for the General Welfare by Establishing a System of Federal Old-Age Benefits, . . . to Establish a Social Security Board; etc. Seventy-fourth Cong., 1st Sess. Cong. Rec. 79(5):5079, 4 April 1935.
122. Debate on Social Security Act. Seventy-fourth Cong., 1st Sess. Cong. Rec. 79(6):6069-6070, 19 April 1935.
123. An Act to Provide for the General Welfare by Establishing a System of Federal Old-Age Benefits. . . ; to Establish a Social Security

Board; etc. Seventy-fourth Cong., 1st Sess. Pub. Stat. at Large U.S. 49(1):620-648, 14 August 1935.
124. Interaction between the A.M.A. and the Committee on Economic Security is described in detail in a memoir by Edwin Witte, Executive Director of the Committee. Witte, Edwin E.: Development of Social Security Act. Madison: University of Wisconsin Press, 1962.
125. Article I, Section 8, (1): The Congress shall have the power to lay and collect taxes . . . , to pay the debts and provide for the common defense and general welfare of the United States. . .
126. Steward Machine Co. *vs.* Davis, Collector of Internal Revenue. United States Reports 301:548-618, 24 May 1937.
127. "The powers not delegated to the United States by the Constitution, nor prohibited by it to the States, are reserved to the States respectively, or to the people."
128. Helvering, Commissioner of Internal Revenue, *et al. vs.* Davis. United States Reports 301:619-646, 24 May 1937.
129. Minutes of House of Delegates: Report of Reference Committee on Consideration of the National Health Program. JAMA 111:1215-1217, 24 September 1938.
130. Editorial: Evidently Change Is Needed. New York Times, 7 February 1921, p. 10.
131. Harding, T. Swann: How Scientific Are Our Doctors? Forum 81:345-351, June, 1929.
132. Rorty, James: Whose Medicine? Nation 143:42-44, 11 July 1936.
133. Rorty, James: Medicine's Misalliance. Nation 146:666-669, 11 June 1938.
134. The American Medical Association. Fortune 18:88-92, 150, 152, 156, 160, 162, 164, 166, 168, November, 1938.
135. Stephenson, H.: Revolt in the AMA. Current History 48:24-26, June, 1938.
136. Arnold, T.: Department of Justice: Statement About Group Health Insurance Case. Current History 49:49-50, September 1938.
137. Minutes of House of Delegates: Report of Board of Trustees. JAMA 116:2791-2792, 21 June 1941.
138. United States *vs.* American Medical Assn., *et al.:* U.S. Court of Appeals for the District of Columbia. No. 7488. Federal Reporter, Series 2 110:703-716, 4 March 1940.
139. Morgan, Hugh J.: Professio. Ann. Int. Med. 28:887-891. May, 1948.
140. Robert Ferdinand Wagner (1877-1953) was born in Germany and came to the United States at an early age. He and Franklin Roosevelt were elected to the New York State Senate about the same time (1910). Wagner served in the U.S. Senate from 1927 to 1949 and was one of the New Deal's staunchest supporters.

141. National Health Act of 1939 (S.1620). Seventy-sixth Cong., 1st Sess. Cong. Rec. 84(2):1976-1982, 28 February 1939.
142. Minutes of House of Delegates: Report of Reference Committee on Consideration of Wagner National Health Bill [17 May]. JAMA 112:2295-2297, 3 June 1939.
143. Social Security Act Amendment of 1943. United National Social Insurance (S.1161). Seventy-eighth Cong., 1st Sess. Cong. Rec. 89(4):5260-5262, 3 June 1943.
144. Editorial: Wagner-Murray-Dingell Bill for Social Security. JAMA 122:600-601, 26 June 1943.
145. Editorial: Does the United States Need a Medical Revolution? JAMA 123:418, 16 October 1943.
146. Editorial: Does Medical Education Need to Be Revolutionized? JAMA 123:484, 23 October 1943
147. Roosevelt, Franklin D.: Message From the President of the United States on the State of the Union. Seventy-eighth Cong., 2nd Sess. Cong. Rec. 90(1):55-57, 11 January 1944, p. 57.
148. Social Security Amendments of 1945 (S.1050). Seventy-ninth Cong., 1st Sess. Cong. Rec. 91(4):4920-4927, 24 May 1945.
149. Editorial: The Wagner-Murray-Dingell Bill (S.1050) of 1945. JAMA 128:364-365, 2 June 1945.
150. Wagner, Robert F.: The Wagner-Murray-Dingell Bill [Letter to the Editor]. JAMA 128:461, 9 June 1945.
151. The Wagner-Murray-Dingell Bill. Senator Wagner Comments on the Journal Editorial. . . . JAMA 128:672-673, 30 June 1945.
152. Editorial: Senator Wagner's Comments. JAMA 128:667-668, 30 June 1945.
153. A Bill . . . to Authorize Grants to the States for Surveying Their Hospitals . . . and for Planning Construction of Additional Facilities, and to Authorize Grants to Assist in Such Construction . . . (S.191). Seventy-ninth Cong., 1st Sess. Cong. Rec. 91(1):158, 10 January 1945.
154. Minutes of House of Delegates: Report of Reference Committee on Legislation and Public Relations. JAMA 129:1200-1201, 22 December 1945.
155. An Act to Amend the Public Health Service Act to Authorize Grants to the States for Surveying Their Hospitals . . . and for Planning Construction of Additional Facilities, and to Authorize Grants to Assist in Such Construction (P.L.79-725). Seventy-ninth Cong., 2nd Sess. Pub. Stat. at Large U.S. 60(1):1040-1049, 13 August 1946.
156. National Health Act of 1945 (S.1606). Seventy-ninth Cong., 1st Sess. Cong. Rec. 91(8):10793-10795, 19 November 1945.
157. Editorial: Senate Hearings on the National Health Program. JAMA 130:1016, 13 April 1946.

158. Editorial: The Hearings on the Wagner-Murray-Dingell Bill. JAMA 131:1424, 24 August 1946.
159. National Health Insurance and Public Health Act (S.1320). Eightieth Cong., 1st Sess. Cong. Rec. 93(4):5516-5522, 20 May 1947.
160. Editorial: Mr. Ewing's Ten Year Health Program. JAMA 138:297-298, 25 September 1947.
161. Minutes of House of Delegates: Report of Reference Committee on Legislation and Public Relations [1 December 1948] JAMA 138:1241, 25 December 1948.
162. Baxter, Leone: Address to House of Delegates. JAMA 140:694-696, 25 June 1949.
163. Minutes of House of Delegates: Statement of Policy of American Medical Association. JAMA 138:1171, 18 December 1948.
164. A Bill to Provide a National Health Insurance and Public Health Program (S.5). Eighty-first Cong., 1st Sess. Cong. Rec. 95(1):38, 5 January 1949.
165. A Bill to Provide a Program of National Health Insurance and Public Health and to Assist in Increasing the Number of Adequately Trained Professional and Other Health Personnel (S.1679). Eighty-first Cong., 1st Sess. Cong. Rec. 95(4):4946, 4959-4962, 25 April 1949.
166. Washington Letter: Compulsory Insurance Chief Issue as Hearings Open. JAMA 140:481-482, 4 June 1949. Editorial: Hearings on Health Legislation. JAMA 140:962, 16 July 1949.
167. It was at this juncture that the faithful and indefatigable Dr. Morris Fishbein, for years editor of the *Journal* and a major spokesman for the A.M.A., was fired. "For thirty-seven years he had been crying 'wolf,' " said Milton Mayer. "Now," Mayer continued, "he was blamed for bringing on the wolves and was thrown to them." (Mayer, Milton: The Rise and Fall of Dr. Fishbein. Harper's Magazine 199:76-85, November, 1949.)
168. The President's Page [Louis H. Bauer]: The Chicago Meeting. JAMA 149:843, 28 June 1952.
169. A Bill to Provide a Program of National Health Insurance and Public Health, etc. (H.R.1817). Eighty-third Cong., 1st Sess. Cong. Rec. 99(1):434, 16 January 1953.
170. Hobby, Oveta Culp: Address of HEW Secretary Before House of Delegates, AMA. JAMA 156:1506-1508, 18 December 1954.
171. Organization Section: Legislative Review. JAMA 156:1514, 18 December 1954.

Several years earlier, an exasperated Congressman, Andrew Biemiller of Wisconsin, had said for the record: "Apparently the only kind of medical aid bill the A.M.A. would approve is a measure which would place unlimited public funds in the hands of the A.M.A. itself, to dispense as it sees fit after paying its lobbying and propaganda

expenses. . . ." (American Medical Association Opposes All Progressive Legislation. New Rival for NAM. Eighty-first Cong., 2nd Sess. Cong. Rec. 96(10):13904-13918, 30 August 1950.)
172. An Act to Provide Medical Care for Dependents of Members of the Uniformed Services, and for Other Purposes (P.L.84-569). Eighty-fourth Cong., 2nd Sess. Pub. Stat. at Large U.S. 70:250-254, 7 June 1956.
173. Editorial: Morale and Medicine. JAMA 163:119, 12 January 1957.
174. A Bill to Amend the Social Security Act . . . so as to Increase the Benefits Payable Under the Federal Old-Age, Survivors, and Disability Insurance Program, to Provide Insurance Against the Costs of Hospital, Nursing Home, and Surgical Services, etc. (H.R.9467). Eighty-fifth Cong., 1st Sess. Cong. Rec. 103(12):16173, 27 August 1957.
175. An Act to Extend and Improve Coverage under the Federal Old-Age, Survivors and Disability Insurance System . . . ; to Provide Grants to the States for Medical Care for Aged Individuals of Low Income; . . . etc. (P.L.86-778). Eighty-sixth Cong., 2nd Sess. Pub. Stat. at Large U.S. 74:924-997, 13 September 1960.
176. A Bill to Provide for Payment for Hospital Services, Skilled Nursing Home Services, and Home Health Services Furnished to Aged Beneficiaries Under the Old-Age Survivors and Disability Insurance Program (H.R.4222). Eighty-seventh Cong., 1st Sess. Cong. Rec. 107(2):2136, 13 February 1961.
177. Medical News: Delegates Endorse Kerr-Mills and AMPAC, Criticize "Public Airing of Disagreements." JAMA 178(11):31, 16 December 1961.
178. Kihss, Peter: A.M.A. Rebuttal to Kennedy Sees Aged Care Hoax. New York Times, 22 May 1962, p. 1.
179. Public Welfare Amendments of 1962 (H.R.10606). Eighty-seventh Cong., 2nd Sess. Cong. Rec. 108(10):13848-13873, 17 July 1962.
180. Social Security Amendments of 1964. Gore Amendment (No. 1256). Eighty-eighth Cong., 2nd Sess. Cong. Rec. 110(16):21113-21122, 31 August 1964.
181. Social Security Amendments of 1964 (H.R.11865). Eighty-eighth Cong., 2nd Sess. Cong. Rec. 110(16):21351-21354, 2 September 1964.
182. A Bill to Amend Titles I and XVI of the Social Security Act to . . . [Authorize] Any State to Provide Medical Assistance for the Aged . . . Under Voluntary Private Health Insurance Plans and to Amend the Internal Revenue Code of 1954 to Provide Tax Incentives to Encourage Prepayment Health Insurance for thy Aged . . . (S.820). Eighty-ninth Cong., 1st Sess. Cong. Rec. 111(2):1461, 28 January 1965.
183. An Act to Provide a Hospital Insurance Program for the Aged Under the Social Security Act With a Supplementary Benefits Program and an Expanded Program of Medical Assistance. . . . etc. Eighty-ninth Cong., 1st Sess. Pub. Stat. at Large U.S. 79:286-423, 30 July 1965.

184. Mills' reasoning, and the means by which the successful Medicare proposal was put together, are described in detail by Harold B. Meyers. The compromise is said to have crystallized in a conference between Mills and Secretary Wilbur Cohen of HEW in March, 1965. (Meyers, Harold B.: Mr. Mills' Elder-medi-better Care. Fortune 71:166-168, 196, June, 1965.)
185. Ward, Donovan F.: Remarks of the President [20 June 1965]. JAMA 193:23-25, 5 July 1965.
186. Appel, James Z.: Inaugural Address. We the People of the United States—Are We Sheep? [20 June 1965]. JAMA 193:26-30, 5 July 1965.
187. Special Announcement: Board of Trustees Action. JAMA 193:689, 23 August 1965.
188. Wilbur, Dwight, L.: Emphasize Steering Instead of the Brake. Inaugural Address. JAMA 205:89-91, 8 July 1968.
189. Hyde, David R.; Wolff, Payson; Gross, Anne; and Hoffman, Elliott Lee: The American Medical Association: Power, Purpose, and Politics in Organized Medicine. Yale Law J. 63:937-1022, May, 1954.
190. Garceau, Oliver: The Political Life of the American Medical Association. Cambridge: Harvard University Press, 1941.
191. Burrow, James G.: A.M.A. Voice of American Medicine. Baltimore: Johns Hopkins Press, 1963.
192. Rayack, Elton: Professional Power and American Medicine: The Economics of ths American Medical Association. Cleveland: World Publishing Company, 1967.
193. Greely, Horace Jr., M.D.: Letter to the Editor. Amer. Med. News 12:5, 3 November 1969.
194. National Health Care—The Gathering Storm. Amer. Med. News 12:1; 8-9, 27 October 1969.
195. Watt, Linda: NHI is Nigh. Today's Health 48:26-29; 71, July, 1970.
196. Forty per cent would come fromfederal tax revenues, 35 per cent from a tax on employer payrolls, and 25 per cent from a tax on individual adjusted gross income.
197. Committee for National Health Insurance: Press Release. Washington, D.C., 7 July 1970.
198. Washington Rounds. Med. World News 11:10f, 19 June 1970.
199. A.M.A. 70. Med. World News 11:19-21, 10 July 1970.

CHAPTER 6

THE FEE-FOR-SERVICE SYSTEM

AN ETHICAL DILEMMA FOR THE MEDICAL PROFESSION

H. Roy Kaplan

The prevailing method of payment for health care in the United States is known as fee-for-service, which means that the recipient of services pays the practitioner or facility directly (or indirectly through a third party) for the services rendered to him. This method of reimbursement for health care may be traced to the Code of Hammurabi which fixed fees according to the status of the patient and his ability to pay.[1] The institutionalization of the fee-for-service system of payment in the United States is, however, derived from two historical trends, one secular and one religious. The first was the organization of business firms into bureaucracies, with rationalization of labor to promote efficiency. This evolved from the free-enterprise system and laissez-faire capitalism which encouraged individual initiative and marketplace behavior in most monetary transactions. The second, religious trend provided the moral underpinning for capitalism and its attendant values, as the famous German sociologist Max Weber has shown.[2] It developed from ascetic Protestantism, with its emphasis on wordly success through individual initiative and work. The Calvinist belief in thrift, deferred gratification, and the moral obligation to work led to the formation of a pervasive work ethic in the West which still occupies an important place in the American value system.[3] Vestiges of this ethic appear in the popular belief that a man should not only work and enjoy it, but that his toil entitles him to the "fruits of his labor." This attitude is often expressed by public officials and "concerned" citizens in denouncing supposed welfare abuses, for many people believe that "he who doesn't work should starve."[4]

While the free enterprise system has produced enormous wealth in our country, it is debatable whether all, or even most, exchange arrangements should be conducted like business transactions. Such a practice is particularly questionable in the field of health care in the United States, where inequities in the distribution of wealth, practitioners, and facilities have contributed to deficiencies in the health of our populace and are placing quality care out of the reach of increasing numbers of persons. In our country, it is generally believed that high cost is synonymous with high quality. We spend more on health care than any other country in the world—approximately 75 billion dollars in fiscal 1971. Yet, for all this expense we are not getting the return that one would expect. In 1967, among 22 industrial countries, United States males ranked 19th in life expectancy, and females sixth.[5] Our infant mortality rate is approximately 20 per thousand, and although this figure is declining, we still rank 15th among industrialized nations and are far behind such countries as Sweden (12.9 per thousand) and Japan (15.3 per thousand).[6] We are the only industrialized nation that does not have a government-sponsored low-cost comprehensive health-care program.

Despite the facade of abundance, all is not well in our society, and, as the data above seem to indicate, our health-care system is suffering severely. The purpose of this paper is to outline some of the ethical and moral dilemmas that arise for health practitioners in their dealings with consumers of health care, especially the poor. These problems may be attributed to the business orientation upon which our system of care is predicated.

The Impact of the Fee-for-Service System on Health Care Practitioners

The ethical problems associated with a fee-for-service system are derived from the nature of the health professions as service-dispensing vocations.[7] Service to the client is the core principle of professionalism,[8] yet this principle is constantly compromised by the fee-for-service system, which is governed by marketplace principles based upon an opposing set of values. As T. H. Marshall noted, the "essence of professionalism" is that "it is not concerned with self-interest but with the welfare of the client."[9] To this end, personal gain and profit must be subordinated to the delivery of the best possible care to the patient. In the professions, the emphasis is on doing a job to the best of one's ability, and matters such as "personal friendship, money, the ethnicity, religion, race, or social class of the client are assumed to be irrelevant."[10] The client's interest must reign supreme and commercialism must be shunned. As Marshall stated: "The professional man, it has been said, does not work in order to be paid: he is paid in order that he may work. Every decision he takes in the course of his career is based on his sense of what is right, not on his estimate of what is profitable."[11]

This lack of mercenary interest has the positive function of creating a bond of trust between the patient and the health practitioner. Without the knowledge that the practitioner has no pecuniary interest in his illness the patient might be unwilling to reveal the extent of his medical problems, or he might hesitate to seek the help of a health professional altogether. Furthermore, since the nature of the service rendered by the medical practitioner is of a highly technical kind, the patient must leave his treatment to his discretion. Professional service is not standardized but is unique to each patient's problems. Marshall notes that unlike the business world where "the commodity can be inspected before it is paid for, the service cannot be . . . The principle of *caveat emptor* is at least plausible when you are buying a horse or a pound of strawberries: It makes nonsense when you are calling in a surgeon to a case of acute appendicitis."[12]

Although these principles are admirable they are frequently compromised by the fee-for-service system. Designed to work most effectively in a state of relative equality, the principles of professionalism have become particularly strained among health practitioners in our society, where inequality in the distribution of means and access to health care is pervasive. In our system, the care given a patient is frequently tied to his ability to pay rather than his need—witness the preoccupation of some hospitals with admitting insured persons. But similar economic considerations also enter into the decision-making of physicians, who must often consider the financial status of patients when prescribing medicines and rendering care. For example, it has been estimated that thousands of lives could be saved in the United States if more funds were available for the use of hemodialysis machines. Undoubtedly, many physicians are prevented from securing this service for patients who need it.[13]

The business orientation directly contravenes the traditionally sacrosanct professional value of monetary disinterestedness. Over four-fifths of the clinical physicians and 90 per cent of the dentists in this country operate their practices in traditional entrepreneurial fashion as solo fee-for-service practitioners. *Medical Economics,* which is received gratis by physicians in the United States, takes pride in displaying the hourly and yearly earnings of physicians by specialties, and average issues contain prescriptions on "How to Reward a Potential Partner's Zeal," "The Fine Art of Heading Off House Calls," "Writing Out the Fee Isn't Enough," "How to Tell if You Need a Business Manager," and "A Tax Free Haven for Your Cash Reserves."[14] While the journal is not an official organ of any medical association, its editors boast of a huge following among physicians. The avid interest of physicians in material drawn from issues of the journal and published as books indicates the business orientation of many health professionals. For example, the *Tax-Savings Guide for Physicians* has sold over 25 thousand copies, and a recent volume entitled *Personal Money Management for Physicians* rivals current best sellers and, according to the editors of the journal, "has outsold several books on our list that have been moving well for years and still are." Among the latter are *Medical Practice Management* and *Medical Partnership Practice.*[15]

Of course we realize that physicians and other health professionals must be paid, but Marshall's admonitions appear to have fallen by the wayside in the hectic confusion of our medical marketplace. (Marshall also emphasizes that the professional man should acquire money legitimately "without impairing the quality of his work or withholding those extra personal services which cannot be specifically demanded by the client and are not specifically paid for."[16])

In 1969, private citizens in this country spent 11.9 billion dollars for physicians' fees—for nearly one-fourth of all personal health-care expenses.[17] While not all physicians are entirely motivated in their practice by monetary incentives, some have exploited the system and their patients. There is evidence that some physicians greatly increased their rates shortly after Medicare was passed. Often charging as much as the system would bear, and in some cases exceeding the reasonable costs established for various types of care, they passed this additional expense on to their elderly and frequently indigent patients.[18] Although we are loath to impute opportunism and unprofessional conduct to these practitioners, such actions cannot be dismissed lightly.

A study by the Medical Disciplinary Committee of the American Medical Association found that overcharging was one of the major problems requiring disciplinary action by state and county medical societies.[19] In discussing the role of discipline in medicine, the committee said:

> . . .what then are the deficiencies which exist within organized medicine—medical societies and specialty groups? First and foremost, the committee found apathy, substantial ignorance, and a lack of a sense of individual responsibility by physicians as a whole. The latter is demonstrated by the "hear no evil, see no evil" attitude of many doctors and through the complaints which are received concerning physicians when the complaining physician later refuses to testify or give a deposition. Without such cooperation the boards and societies are powerless to act.[20]

Despite the emphasis on disregard for monetary recompense in the health professional's code of ethics, he is frequently forced into compromising situations which threaten the moral fabric of his profession. Physicians in solo practice must make considerable investments for office space and equipment and frequently pass on these expenditures to their patients in the form of increased fees. Although there is nothing immoral about this activity in the business world, such practices seem inconsistent with the professional service ethic.

Furthermore, evaluating the financial status of patients not only appears to violate the professional's tenet of monetary disinterestedness, but reinforces his entrepreneurial role. Frequently, physicians are cast in the role of clerk and bill collector, and often secure the services of agencies for this purpose when patients are recalcitrant.

Further pressures exerted by the marketplace on the behavior of health professionals are apparent in the geographical distribution of practitioners in the United States. While approximately 25 per cent of our population lives in rural areas, only 12 per cent of our physicians, 18 per cent of our nurses, 14 per cent of our pharmacists, 8 per cent of our pediatricians, and less than 4 per cent of our psychiatrists are located there.[21] A recent study by the American Medical Association revealed that the 300 Standard Metropolitan Statistical Areas in the United States contained 85.2 per cent of the non-federally employed physicians. It also reported the tendency of specialists to congregate in urban areas, while general practitioners were more frequently located in less densely populated places.[22] But a maldistribution of health professionals exists even in urban areas, with wealthy sections having a disproportionate share of medical practitioners and facilities. Venice, a Los Angeles community, has more than 60 thousand persons and a physician-population ratio of nine per 100 thousand compared to a ratio of 125 per 100 thousand in Los Angeles County as a whole, and 1,800 per 100 thousand in Beverly Hills.[23] The Bronx provides us with another example. Dr. Harold B. Wise, director of the Montefiore Hospital Neighborhood Medical Care Demonstration Project, has noted the discrepancy:

> A major problem that has been discussed is the lack of medical manpower in this area. In these 55 blocks that we live in, there used to be 25 doctors practicing, now there are four. There used to be only 25 thousand people living here and now there are close to

> 50 thousand. So in the Bronx where you have one doctor for 700 people, in this part of the Bronx you have one doctor for 10 thousand people.[24]

Among the factors operating to produce this lopsided self-segregation of physicians, and particularly of specialists in urban areas, are the desire to practice medicine in places that have sufficient medical facilities such as laboratories and hospitals; the opportunity to associate with one's colleagues and to continue one's education; and the tendency to establish a practice in the vicinity where one graduated from medical school. But economic motivations should not be discounted. The number of physicians per 100 thousand of population closely corresponds to the per-capita income of the residents for any region of the United States.[25] As long as these factors are paramount in the decision-making process governing the distribution of health resources, we will have a self-perpetuating cycle in which poverty and the lack of health resources contribute to the maldistribution of health personnel and facilities.

A study conducted among American physicians and British physicians employed in the National Health Service revealed a higher degree of patient-centered service orientation among the British practitioners. The British doctors evinced satisfaction with many aspects of their system including the freedom they had to dispense the care their patients needed without having to worry about their financial means, and the freedom of patients to seek treatment irrespective of cost. They also expressed satisfaction with the removal of billing responsibilities, which they considered time-consuming and essentially unrelated to their professional tasks. Their American counterparts stressed the freedom they enjoyed under the capitalist system and the competitive aspects of working in a free market. The investigator concluded that British physicians manifested higher degrees of professionalism, particularly with respect to the service norm.[26] This research can be viewed as evidence of the perverting influence that the fee-for service system has had upon professional behavior in the United States.

Clearly the fee-for-service system is an unhealthy milieu for the health professionals healing functions. By linking illness with remuneration, the fee-for-service system focuses health professionals' and patients' attention on sickness rather than on disease prevention, and theoretically, if not always in actuality, gives medical practitioners a vested interest in morbidity. And the chief spokesman of the medical profession in the United States, the American Medical Association, has not seen fit to rectify this situation. Indeed, while it was founded "to promote the science and art of medicine and the betterment of public health," its record of achievements in the latter area is less than enviable, as several authors have shown.[27] In its zeal to keep medicine in the fold of the free enterprise system and protect physicians from third-party interference in their practice, the A.M.A., as Harris notes, opposed compulsory vaccinations against smallpox and compulsory inoculations against diphtheria, the mandatory reporting of tuberculosis cases to public health agencies, the establishment of public venereal-disease clinics and Red Cross blood banks, federal grants for construction of medical schools and scholarships for medical students, and free centers for cancer diagnosis.[28] The A.M.A. spent millions of dollars in its fight to prevent the passage of various forms of compulsory government health insurance. Today it is adopting a more moderate attitude, but its Medicredit proposal for health-care payments, which has been presented to Congress for consideration, is still predicated upon traditional free-enterprise principles which emphasize individual initiative and responsibility in matters pertaining to health-care fees, and "cost consciousness" on the part of health-care consumers. As late as 1969, the House of Delegates of the A.M.A. stated that "private practice remains the best method of serving mankind's medical needs."[29]

The spread of group practice among health practitioners in this country has been hailed as a significant step toward removing some of the practitioners' burdens while improving the quality of care to patients. There is much to be said for such pooling of resources and sharing of income. However, not all groups operate on this basis, some preferring instead to be merely convenient business arrangements designed to lessen the work loads of the participants. In these situations the financial incentives to health care persist, and so do the attendant ethical dilemmas. Indeed, even groups that pool revenues may be perpetuating the fee for-service system, unless they operate on a prepaid basis. Perhaps that is why the A.M.A. has reversed its opposition to group practice.[30]

The Effect of the Fee-for-Service System on the Poor

Payment for health care is a problem even for people in prepaid group health insurance plans. Many just cannot meet the cost. This fact leads us into a discussion of the second ethical and moral dilemma stemming from the fee-for-service system: the inequities that it perpetrates on the poor. Medical costs are escalating in this country. While the Consumer Price Index has risen steadily since World War II, medical price increases have far exceeded the other items in the index. Between 1965 and 1968 the cost of medical care increased at an annual rate of 5.8 per cent compared to a 3.3 per cent increase for all other consumer prices.[31] During this same period, daily service charges for hospitals rose at an annual rate of 13.9 per cent, and physicians' fees, which had been increasing by less than 3 per cent annually between 1960 and 1965, jumped to a 6.1 per cent annual increase.[32] It has been estimated that if current rates of growth in our economy continue there will be an increase in total expenditures on health care of nearly 140 per cent by 1975, with physician-directed services rising almost 160 per cent, dentist-directed services increasing almost 65 per cent, and costs of short-term general hospital services 250 per cent. Individual per capita expenditures on health care would then be over 400 dollars and the total national expenditure for health care nearly 100 billion dollars.[33]

Today, even the more affluent can hardly afford to become ill. In the face of such monumental costs it is not difficult to understand why illness plays havoc with the poor; their economic predicament often leaves them unprepared or unable to cope with it. Since the costs of physician and hospital services are high, and the poor are seldom insured for such contingencies (only 34 per cent of families earning less than two thousand dollars a year have health insurance compared to 90 per cent of the population with incomes of seven thousand dollars or more),[34] it becomes an ethical imperative to remove the economic obstacles which impede access to quality health care for all Americans. Few of the 30 to 40 million disadvantaged members of our society, whose ranks are swollen in times of economic recession, can afford adequate health care, since for them, and many others, illness is rapidly "pricing itself out of the free marketplace."[35] Consequently, the poor frequently resort to quacks and folk remedies, and their medicine chests often contain such items as kidney and liver pills, stomach tonics, and blood builders.[36] As one writer concludes, " 'Lower-class' life is crisis-life, constantly trying to 'make do' with string where rope is needed."[37]

The effects of high health care costs, combined with shortages and maldistributions of health personnel and facilities, have adversely affected the health of a substantial proportion of our population. This can be viewed as a concomitant result of the institutionalization of the fee-for-service system, which had not undergone any major changes from its business orientation in the last hundred years until the passage in 1965 of Public Law 89-97 with its provisions for medical care for the elderly and the indigent. Despite this legislation, which Chapman and Talmadge elsewhere in this volume see as evidence of the belief in the right to health in the United States, disparities in the quality and amount of health care received by disadvantaged members of our society persist.

In general, the following people are the recipients of inadequate health care, sharing a common bond of poverty and ill health: persons who reside in rural areas, members of minority groups (especially nonwhites), and the aged.

Rural Poor. The laws of supply and demand,when applied to the availability and reception of health care, have been particularly onerous on the rural poor. Poverty is rampant in rural America. Proportionately twice as many people are poor in rural areas as in urban ones, and 75 per cent of the rural poor are white.[38] The plight of the rural poor is complicated by their residence in places which do not have sufficient quality health manpower and facilities; even if they had the money to pay, they would still be hard put to obtain service. Despite the existence of a comparable number of hospital beds between urban and rural areas, there are no hospital facilities of 25 beds or more within a 25-mile distance of over four million Americans, and approximately 200 thousand people live over 50 miles away from such facilities.[39] But these figures are somewhat misleading when we consider that hospitals having less than 100 beds are generally presumed to be too small to offer optimal health care; hence, the number of people living great distances from quality facilities is probably much larger.

The disproportionate share of health personnel and facilities in rural areas has, as we previously noted, made them medically deprived. Statistics demonstrating the cumulative effect of geographical segregation illustrate this deprivation. For example, in 1969 there were 234 physicians per 100 thousand people in New York and 78 per 100 thousand in Mississippi and Alaska. While there were 61 dentists per 100 thousand persons in Massachusetts, South Carolina had only 22 for the same number of people.[40]

The low per-capita income of rural residents also appears to limit the number of times they see a physician. During fiscal 1966-67 the number of physician visits was lowest among persons living on farms, and this was particularly pronounced among children living in the South.[41] Like the majority of medically deprived persons, rural residents frequently lack knowledge about preventive medicine. This situation may be complicated by the absence of any public health agency that could provide information and services pertaining to immunization from disease. The consequences of these deficiencies are manifested in the high rates of infant and maternal mortality in rural areas. One-third of the maternal mortality in 1964 was in rural areas and small towns of less than 10 thousand people.[42]

The inferior health status of American Indians provides us with a vivid illustration of how one segment of the rural population fares under our system of marketplace medicine. In the past, infant mortality among Indians was considerably more than twice that among whites. Although this has been reduced, it is still far above the national average. Most infant deaths among Indians are the result of respiratory conditions, gastroenteritis, and diarrheas. In fact, nearly one-sixth of *all* Indian deaths in a year are the result of tuberculosis and of gastroenteric and other infectious diseases.[43]

After reviewing the health problems of low income people in rural America, the President's National Advisory Commission on Rural Poverty concluded, "Nowhere in the United States is the need for health services so acute, and nowhere is it so inadequate."[44]

Nonwhites. One does not have to live in a rural area to be medically needy. The desperately bad health status of nonwhites, especially blacks, is graphically illustrated by their high rates of maternal and infant mortality. As with the Indians, the black infant mortality rate of 32.5 per thousand in 1970 was approximately twice that of the white (18 per thousand), and this disparity has shown signs of increasing. In 1945-46 the nonwhite to white differential in infant mortality rates was 1.6 to one, but it had risen to 1.9 to one by 1963-64. The 11 per cent reduction in mortality of white infants from the years 1953-54 to 1963-64 was twice that of the nonwhites.[45] Apparently these trends are continuing, for the 1970 figures indicate a decline in the white infant death rate of .8 per cent and an *increase* in the nonwhite rate of .2 per cent. A substantial proportion of black infant deaths occur in urban ghettos. For example, the infant mortality rates in black communities in Cleveland are approximately 40 per cent higher than in white communities, with death in the first months of life 70 per cent higher.[46]

Closely paralleling the high rates of infant deaths are those of maternal mortality among nonwhites. In 1967 there was one maternal death in the United States for every 3,500 live births. There was, however a great disparity between the death rates of whites and nonwhites—nonwhite women had a rate almost four times higher than whites, and there is reason to believe that here, too, the differences are increasing.[47] The main cause of these disparities would seem to be the lack of prenatal and postnatal care among nonwhite women, a theory supported by the fact that white women experienced a 40 per cent decline in maternal mortality attributable to sepsis during the decade 1955-65, while nonwhites registered a decline of less than 10 per cent.[48]

Studies conducted by the Metropolitan Life Insurance Company have consistently shown that there are higher rates of mortality from cancer, diabetes, and influenza among lower socioeconomic groups than among the more affluent members of our society, and these rates are particularly accentuated among nonwhites. For example, the death rate among nonwhite females in the United States from uterine malignancies is more than double that among whites, and, coincidentally, well above the rates reported by many Western nations.[49]

The Aged. Our society has more than 20 million persons aged 65 and over and this figure is constantly increasing. However, the incomes of most people are reduced almost to half of what they were before age 65, so that a majority of our elderly citizens are poor. The poverty of the aged hinders their attempts to secure adequate health care, although they are greatly in need of it, for over 80 per cent of persons 65 and older have one or more chronic health conditions which limit their ability to perform their normal daily activities.[50] The increased need of health care among the elderly is reflected in their larger proportion of physician visits compared to the rest of the population,[51] and in their increased drug consumption. In 1968, the per-capita cost of prescribed medicines for persons under 65 was 14.54 dollars, but it was 40.69 dollars for persons 65 and over.[52]

The escalation of health-care costs, the decline in the number of physicians in general practice, and the decreasing number of house calls made by physicians pose serious threats to the physical and mental well-being of the elderly. At present, Medicare meets only 45 per cent of their total health-care expenditures, and our senior citizens are left to fend for themselves in the chaos of the medical marketplace. In medical shortage areas, where health personnel and facilities are lacking, an aged person must provide his own transportation to and from a practitioner or an institution often at great discomfort, inconvenience, and cost. The following story of one patient is a heartrending account of some problems that may confront the elderly in this country.

> May I take the time of a distinguished committee of the U.S. Senate to tell of one aged patient who, like most old people, suffered from multiple diagnoses? He had a serious eye problem—actually two diseases: glaucoma and keratitis—for which he received care at a nearby medical center, in the department of opthalmology. His personal doctor, a good internist, however, had diagnosed a mild diabetes, and for this periodic visits were necessary to an office eight miles away. Painful corns and bunions, impairing the ability to walk, were not within the specialty of the personal doctor, so these required periodic visits to a podiatrist at an office six miles in another direction. Dental care, in an effort to save the few remaining teeth, so that dentures would fit more firmly and food could be more properly chewed, required numerous visits to a dentist at still another location.
>
> Then a bladder problem developed and prostatic disease was suspected. At about the same period, the patient showed lethargy and confusion, suggesting a mild cerebrovascular accident. The personal doctor made a home call and the decision was to hospitalize. A bed was not immediately available—except in a small proprietary hospital which the family refused—and it was not till 10 days later that he could be admitted to a good voluntary general hospital 15 miles away. After X-rays, cystoscopy, and other examinations there, his treatment was stabilized. In the workup, it was discovered that a drug the opthalmologist had been prescribing for many months was causing serious side effects, which had been missed by the internist since these two specialists had never communicated with each other. The patient was then admitted to a sanatorium, selected for its closeness to the family home, so that visits from the patient's children would be possible daily. This was one of the "better" nursing homes—it was certainly expensive enough at 32 dollars a day paid by Medicare—but this was evidently not costly enough to support a proper staff. After a few days, because of the lack of proper surveillance, this aged patient was found roaming on the street.

When this happened a second time, the commercial proprietor decided to discharge the patient as "too difficult to care for." It took five weeks of nursing care at home, with daily problems of incontinence of urine and feces, before a bed in another nursing home became available.

The latter facility proved to be better managed and the patient improved. After only two weeks, however, he was getting up from a chair one day, when he fell and fractured his left hip. This required an orthopedic surgeon, readmission to the hospital, and preparation for a major operation. But then complications to the diabetes set in, because of the traumatic shock of fracture. A delay over 24 hours in reporting a critical laboratory test nearly cost the patient's life at this time. Had the hospital been adequately staffed, this delay would not have occurred. A skillful operation, with a pinning of the broken bone, was done. Special-duty nurses costing 111 dollars per day—over and above the Medicare coverage of the hospital bill—had to be hired because of the shortage of regular hospital nurses.

I have not recounted the other details of multiple drug prescriptions, special services of an appliance shop to adjust the bed at home, the physical therapy required for a knee injury, and much more. This patient was my widowed father, who lived with my wife and me for nine years after his retirement from 51 years of medical practice. My abbreviated account of his medical care problems applies only to the last year, or it would be much longer. Accounts like this could be told thousands of times over, each day in the United States, and would doubtless be more complex and disturbing for a family less well informed about the jungle of medical care delivery.

I was notified by telephone when I arrived in Washington late last night that my father had just died.[53]

Where is the morality in a society which forces its elderly citizens into retirement, robbing them of meaningful activities, and then makes inadequate provisions for the health care that would enable them to engage in viable substitutes? Is there equity in the myriad private health plans which drop aged persons like hot potatoes when they miss premium payments? Is there justice in a system which compels some disoriented elderly persons to make decisions regarding vital health matters in the same manner as they would buy food at a supermarket?

Other Obstacles Impeding Adequate Health Care

Various cultural and environmental barriers impede the effective delivery of quality health care to some persons in the United States, and Rosenblatt has identified several of these among the urban poor; for example, their lack of familiarity with organized health systems and the impersonality of bureaucratic health-care organizations.[54] Clinics in poor areas are frequently understaffed and overcrowded, with long waiting periods for people seeking treatment. It is not uncommon for a person to receive treatment from a different physician each time he goes to a clinic, further adding to the impersonal atmosphere of the surroundings and increasing the possibility of inferior care in cases where insufficient information may be recorded by staff who are overburdened with heavy caseloads. This difficulty is in addition to the spiraling increase in the cost of health care and its attendant anomalies in the distribution of health personnel and facilities.

Confronted with these impediments to better health, there is little wonder that many Americans, especially the poor, frequently do not practice preventive health care. This is particularly apparent with reference to dental care. In the Health Examination Survey conducted between 1960 and 1962, it was found that more than 20 million persons had lost all their teeth, and an additional 10 million had lost all 16 teeth in either the upper or lower jaw; and the number of endentulous persons increased sharply with advancing age.[55] The National Health Survey of 1963-64 revealed that almost 17 per cent of the population had never been to a dentist.[56]

During fiscal 1966-67, 36.2 per cent of families whose annual incomes were less than 3,000 dollars did not see a physician.[57] The number of physician visits to nonwhites is only half that for whites in the United States, indicating that they do not practice preventive health care to the same extent, and do not receive adequate care.[58] Recent physical examinations given to a group of 630 children from west Harlem who were participating in the summer Fresh Air Fund program for disadvantaged urban youths revealed 835 specific medical problems, including: 248 cases of iron deficiency anemia, 265 kidney ailments, 165 children in need of dental work, 48 in need of eye glasses, 300 afflicted with sickle-cell anemia, 29 with minor tuberculosis, 14 with heart murmurs, 11 with ear problems, five with skin diseases, four with serious respiratory problems, and one with syphilis.[59]

In this country we have a catastrophic orientation to illness and disease. This is encouraged by the fee-for service method of payment, bolstered as it is by the myriad private health (sic) insurance programs, most of which provide little or no incentive or reimbursement for routine preventive care. In their frantic efforts to vie for subscribers, they have left their reimbursement schedules to the exigencies of the marketplace. Approximately 60 per cent of the increases in medical care costs in the last decade were the result of inflation, and the health-insurance industry bears much of the responsibility for this. Blue Cross, which was originally founded to help individuals meet their hospital bills, has become the chief source of income for hospitals and has often abnegated its social and humanitarian goals in favor of serving as the bursar of our fee-for-service system. Blue Cross has promoted much of the increase in hospital costs by running on a cost-plus basis, in essence reimbursing hospitals for services rendered to subscribers without exercising effective controls to insure efficiency.

While nearly four-fifths of the people in the United States have some form of health insurance, many of these persons receive inadequate health care. In 1968-69, private health insurance benefits were meeting only 22 per cent of the total health care expenditures in the United

States.[60] For many people high health insurance premiums place even these insufficient benefits out of reach. The Committee for National Health Insurance estimated that in 1968 24 million people under 65 had no hospital insurance, another 35 million had no surgical insurance of any kind, and 61 million people had no in hospital medical coverage.[61] The *type* of coverage provided by the majority of the health insurance plans is also sorely deficient. Most emphasize in-patient hospital care, which fosters over-utilization and discourages preventive outpatient care by physicians.

Recent attempts by Blue Cross to switch from a community rating procedure for the establishment of reimbursement fees to one predicated upon the health status of the insured has ominous overtones for many Americans, particularly the groups of persons whose health status we discussed. Such a system would be particularly onerous on the poor whose higher rates of illness make them more of a risk and hence would precipitate an increase in their premiums.[62] The fee-for-service system forces individuals and organizations to seek means by which they can maximize profits and minimize losses—a further indication of the disastrous effects that marketplace values can have on our health-care system.[63]

Pay-as-you-go medicine necessarily prevents some people from getting anywhere in their quest for quality health care. But even when some of our disadvantaged citizens desire to obtain health care, they are hindered by our traditional belief in rugged individualism and self-reliance. Some staunch advocates of the work ethic disapprove of programs of "socialized" medicine, and even of some public health legislation. Supporters of this philosophy by and large believe that public welfare programs predicated upon the deliverance of services at little or no cost inhibit individual initiative by giving rewards without "proper" expenditures of energy through work. Implicit in this assumption is the belief that the poor are poor because they have not adequately internalized the work ethic and, consequently, if they know that services will be provided to them irrespective of their life styles, there will no longer be any incentive for them to work. Indeed, some people believe that services should not be provided to the poor because they are poor, which is to say that they do not deserve help because they have not demonstrated their inclination or ability to help themselves. Such positions easily degenerate into social-Darwinistic arguments which attribute poverty exclusively to individual weaknesses rather than recognizing the role of social institutions in its formation and perpetuation.

The net result of such thinking, in addition to denying the efficacy of welfare programs, is the stigmatization of persons who avail themselves of public assistance. When applied to public health care legislation this work ethic yields some interesting disparities. For example, we find the present Administration of our federal government vowing to rectify the inequities in our health care system while simultaneously opposing comprehensive changes in the method of payment on the grounds that it is "alien to our basic traditions."[64]

Vestiges of this conservative philosophy can be found in our public health legislation. For example, Dr. George Reader has noted evidence of the work ethic in the differing eligibility requirements for Medicare and Medicaid.[65] In the former, there is a guaranteed right to medical care for elderly persons signifying they have earned it by reaching a specified age and ostensibly being productive members of our society for many years. Medicaid, however, uses a means test as the criterion for determining eligibility, implying that the poor are not entitled to health care merely because they need it, and must, in effect, humble themselves in order to obtain it. The end result of this policy has been to make some eligible persons reluctant to participate in public welfare programs. Dramatic evidence of the stigma attached to public assistance in the form of Medicaid can be seen in the following remarks of participants in this program in New York:

> I receive Social Security, but I have to have Welfare supplementation. . . I have a friend. . .She's 95 years old and she lives on less than 80 dollars a month. But she won't approach Medicaid because she thinks Welfare means charity. And there is stigma there. [Ellipses in original.]
>
> One thing that did happen the first visit that I went to the dentist. He said, "Oh, are you on Welfare now?" when I showed him the Medicaid card. And I said, "Well, no, that doesn't mean that we're on Welfare. It just happens that that's what it says on the top of the card—Department of Welfare."[66]

Such remarks point up the pervasiveness of the work ethic, for it appears to have been internalized by those persons upon whom it has worked inequities. Since the fee-for-service system is inextricably intertwined with this ethic, it stands to reason that such thinking will impede the delivery and reception of quality health care for the less privileged members of our society. While the virtue of thrift is deeply imbedded in American traditions, frugality in health care, as we have seen, has consistently led to hardship among the less fortunate. Fundamental prerequisites for the delivery of comprehensive quality health care to all Americans must, then, be an alteration of this philosophy and of the present system of reimbursement for health care services. Even in 1951 the editors of the *Annals of the American Academy of Political and Social Science* noted that "the issue is not whether medical care is superior to that in other countries, but whether it is as good as it ought to be in this country with such resources and facilities . . an unparalleled standard of living, and an unalterable belief in equal opportunity."[67]

Of course, we recognize that many problems must be surmounted in order to increase the efficiency and effectiveness of our health-care system. The logistics of rectifying the shortage and maldistribution of health personnel and facilities must be solved, as well as the education of the population in public health and routine preventive health care. But significant changes in the present system will not occur unless we first alter our conception of the utility of free enterprise in medicine. Such a value change will require many Americans to accept that there may well be weaknesses in our present institutional structure. But values change slowly, and such changes often need to be precipitated by some sort of crisis. We are in that crisis now. Whether the change is agreeable to the medical profession and best for the population will depend on how fundamental our desire is to redress the inequities in our health care system. As the richest nation in the world, with a gross national product over a trillion dollars, we have the resources to solve many of the problems related to health care. The American people must decide whether it is not time that we altered our archaic tradition of having sick people compete as consumers in a free market for care. They must consider whether it is not time we stopped letting the free marketplace influence the quality, standards, and delivery of health care in the United States.

References

1. Lyman A. Brewer, "De Humanitate," *American Journal of Surgery*, 118 (August, 1969), p. 134.
2. Max Weber, *The Protestant Ethic and the Spirit of Capitalism*, Talcott Parsons (trans.) (New York: Charles Scribner's Sons, 1958).
3. Robin M. Williams, *American Society: A Sociological Interpretation*, third edition (New York: Alfred A. Knopf, 1970), pp. 458-461; Cora Du Bois, "The Dominant Value Profile of American Culture," *American Anthropologist*, 57 (December, 1955), p. 1234; Robert K. Merton, "Social Structure and Anomie," *Social Theory and Social Structure* (New York: The Free Press, 1968, enlarged edition), p. 193.

4. This often-quoted phrase has a Biblical origin. Paul exhorts the Thessalonians to avoid idleness while waiting for the return of the Savior, for "If any would not work, neither should he eat." The Second Epistle of Paul to the Thessalonians, Chapter 3, Verse 10.

5. "Higher Education and the Nation's Health," *The Carnegie Commission on Higher Education* (October, 1970), p. 14.

6. Ibid., pp. 17-18.

7. Some of the following discussion on professionalism is drawn from the unpublished manuscript "Professionalism" by Professor Bhopinder S. Bolaria, Department of Sociology, University of Saskatchewan, Saskatoon.

8. Harold L. Wilensky, "The Professionalization of Everyone?" *American Journal of Sociology*, 70 (September, 1964), p. 140.

9. T.H. Marshall, "Professionalism and Social Policy," *In Man, Work, and Society*, Sigmund Nosow, William H. Form, eds. (New York: Basic Books, Inc., 1962), p. 226.

10. Edward Gross, *Work and Society* (New York: Thomas Crowell, 1958), p. 79.

11. T. H. Marshall, "The Recent History of Professionalism in Relation to Social Structure and Social Policy," *Canadian Journal of Economics and Political Science*, 5 (1939), p. 325.

12. Marshall, "The Recent History of Professionalism in Relation to Social Structure and Social Policy," *op. cit.*, pp. 327-328.

13. Constantine L. Hampers, Eugene Schupak, *Long-Term Hemodialysis* (New York: Grune and Stratton, 1967), pp.4-8. "Use of Artificial Kidneys Poses Awesome Questions," *New York Times*, October 24, 1971, pp. 1, 57.

14. The first two articles appear in *Medical Economics* (February 3, 1969), and the last three are from the October 13, 1969 issue.

15. *Medical Economics* (October 13, 1969), pp.10-11.

16. Marshall, "The Recent History of Professionalism in Relation to Social Structure and Social Policy," *op. cit.*, p. 331.

17. *The Size and Shape of the Medical Care Dollar*, U. S. Department of Health, Education, and Welfare, Social Security Administration (Washington, D.C.: Government Printing Office, 1970), p. 20.

18. See the statement of New York State Senator Seymour Thaler for supporting evidence in *Costs and Delivery of Health Services to Older Americans*, Part 2, Hearings before the Subcommittee on Health of the Elderly, U. S. Senate (Washington, D.C.: Government Printing Office, 1968), pp. 426-435. Also, in the same volume, see the statement of Walter Newburgher, President of the Congress of Senior Citizens, for additional information on this subject, pp. 460-463. The reader is also referred to Walter K. Emory, "Warning: Medicare Scandals Ahead," *Medical Economics* (May 29, 1967) pp. 141-157.

19. *Report of the Medical Disciplinary Committee to the Board of Trustees*. American Medical Association (June, 1961), p. 9.
20. Ibid., p. 52.
21. "The People Left Behind," *Report of the President's National Advisory Commission on Rural Poverty* (Washington, D. C.: Government Printing Office, 1967), p. 63.
22. J. N. Haug, G. A. Roback, *Distribution of Physicians, Hospitals, and Hospital Beds in the United States, 1967*, Department of Survey Research (Chicago: American Medical Association, 1968), pp. 6-14.
23. Lester Breslow, "The Urgency of Social Action for Health," *American Journal of Public Health*, 60 (January, 1970), p. 12.
24. Statement of Harold B. Wise in *Costs and Delivery of Health Services to Older Americans*, p. 416.
25. Corroborating evidence can be found in "Rurality, Poverty, and Health: Medical Problems in Rural Areas," U. S. Department of Agriculture, Agricultural Economic Report No. 172 (Washington, D.C.: Government Printing Office, February, 1970), pp. 5-6, especially table 4. See also W. G. Rimlinger and H. B. Steele, "Economic Interpretation of the Spatial Distribution of Physicians in the United States," *Southern Economic Journal*, 30 (July, 1963), pp. 1-12. The American Academy of General Practice encourages this phenomenon when it exhorts practitioners to consider the following questions when selecting a location for establishing a practice, "Has the average family income growth been equal to or above average for the state? for the nation? Does the physicians' fee schedule represent change in proportion to other rising costs? Does the average gross and net income of general practitioners in the community compare with like-populated areas in the state?" *Organization and Management of Family Practice*, American Academy of General Practice, Kansas City, Missouri, 1968, pp. 29-30.
26. Bhopinder S. Bolaria, "Professionalism Among American and English Physicians," unpublished doctoral dissertation, Washington State University, 1967, Pullman, Washington.
27. Richard Harris, *A Sacred Trust* (New York: The New American Library, Inc., 1966); Odin W. Anderson, *The Uneasy Equilibrium* (New Haven: College and University Press, 1968); Ed Cray, *In Failing Health* (Indianapolis: The Bobbs-Merrill Company, Inc., 1970); Barbara Ehrenreich, John Ehrenreich, *The American Health Empire: Power, Profits, and Politics* (New York: Vintage Books, 1971).
28. Harris, *op. cit.*, p. 2.
29. The House also established a Committee on Private Practice which was delegated, among other things, to develop new methods to promote private practice throughout medical school, graduate, and post-

graduate training; help the private practitioner improve his methods of providing medical care (including business practices), and publicize the merits of private practice. *Journal of the American Medical Association*, 211 (January 12, 1970) , p. 183.

30. A recent A.M.A. report, *Profile of Medical Practice, 1971*, indicated that doctors in two-man partnerships were earning approximately four thousand dollars more a year than those in solo practice.

31. *The Size and Shape of the Medical Care Dollar*, p. 9.

32. *Ibid.*, p. 10.

33. *Report of the National Advisory Commission on Health Manpower*, November, 1967, Vol. 1 (Washington, D. C.: Government Printing Office, 1967), p. 34.

34. *Report of the National Advisory Commission on Civil Disorders* (Washington, D. C.: Government Printing Office, March 1, 1968), p. 136.

35. Edgar May, *The Wasted Americans* (New York: The New American Library, 1965), p. 97.

36. Robert L. Eichhorn, Edward G. Ludwig, "Poverty and Health," in *Poverty in the Affluent Society*, Hanna M. Meissner, ed. (New York: Harper and Row, Inc., 1966), p. 179.

37. S. M. Miller, "The American Lower Classes: A Typological Approach," *Social Research*, 31 (1964) , p. 13.

38. *Rural Poverty*, Conference Proceedings of the National Association for Community Development, January 30-February 1, 1967 (Washington, D.C.: National Association for Community Development, April, 1967) , p. 1.

39. *Report of the National Advisory Commission on Health Manpower, op. cit.*, p. 37.

40. *Statistical Abstracts of the United States, 1970,* U. S. Bureau of the Census, 91st edition (Washington, D. C.: Government Printing Office, 1970), p. 67.

41. "Volume of Physician Visits: United States—July 1966-June 1967," *Vital and Health Statistics*, Series 10, No. 49 (November, 1968), p. 5.

42. "The People Left Behind," p. 59.

43. *Ibid.*, p. 73.

44. *Ibid.*, p. 59.

45. "Infant Mortality in the United States and Abroad," *Statistical Bulletin of the Metropolitan Life Insurance Company*, 48 (May, 1967), p. 5.

46. "A Time to Listen . . . A Time to Act," *Report of the United States Commission on Civil Rights* (Washington, D. C.: Government Printing Office, November, 1967), p. 21.

47. *Report of the National Advisory Commission on Civil Disorders, op. cit.*, p. 136.

48. "Maternal Mortality in the United States and Abroad," *Statistical Bulletin of the Metropolitan Life Insurance Company*, 49 (December, 1968), p. 5.
49. "Cancer Mortality Trends Among Women in Various Countries," *Statistical Bulletin of the Metropolitan Life Insurance Company*, 48 (December, 1967), p. 9; "Diabetes and Socioeconomic Level," *Statistical Bulletin of the Metropolitan Life Insurance Company*, 49 (August, 1968), pp. 5-7. There is an interesting discussion of the relationship between health and income by Monroe Lerner entitled "Social Differences in Physical Health," in *Poverty and Health: A Sociological Analysis*, John Kosa, *et al.*, (eds.), (Cambridge: Harvard University Press, 1969), pp. 69-112. There is also an extensive review of studies relating to this topic in Patricia A. Leo and George Rosen's article "A Bookshelf on Poverty and Health," *American Journal of Public Health*, 59 (April, 1969), pp. 591-607.
50. "Limitation of Activity and Mobility Due to Chronic Conditions: United States—July 1965-June 1966," *Vital and Health Statistics*, Series 10, No. 45 (Washington, D. C.: Government Printing Office, May, 1968), pp. 6-8.
51. "Volume of Physician Visits . . .", *op. cit.*, pp. 4-5.
52. *Prescription Drug Data Summary*, U. S. Department of Health, Education, and Welfare, Social Security Administration (Washington, D.C.: Government Printing Office, July, 1970), p. 12.
53. Statement of Dr. Milton I. Roemer, M.D. and Professor, School of Public Health, University of California, Los Angeles. Appearing in *Costs and Delivery of Health Services to Older Americans*, Part 1, Hearings before the Subcommittee on Health of the Elderly, U. S. Senate, (Washington, D. C.: Government Printing Office, 1967), pp. 84-85.
54. Daniel Rosenblatt, "Barriers to Medical Care for the Urban Poor," in *New Perspectives on Poverty*, Arthur B. Shostak, William Gomberg, eds. (Englewood Cliffs: Prentice-Hall, Inc., 1965), pp. 69-76.
55. "Selected Dental Findings in Adults by Age, Race, and Sex, United States—1960-1962," *Vital and Health Statistics*, Series 11, No. 7 (November, 1965), pp. 6-7.
56. "Dental Visits: Time Interval Since Last Visit, United States—July 1963-June 1964," *Vital and Health Statistics*, Series 10, No. 29 (April, 1966), p. 1.
57. "Volume of Physician Visits . . ." *op. cit.*, p. 38.
58. *Ibid.*
59. Lacey Fosburgh, "Medical Aid Given by Fresh Air Fund," *New York Times*, June 6, p. 80.
60. "Higher Education and the Nation's Health," p. 20.
61. Cray, *op. cit.*, p. 213.

62. Ehrenreich and Ehrenreich, *op. cit.*, pp. 151-152.
63. Not all insurance programs are afflicted with high degrees of inertia. While Blue Cross and Blue Shield, the largest insurers in the nation, remain fairly adamant toward change, some private companies have developed more innovative and rational approaches aimed at increasing preventive care, e.g., the Kaiser plan which emphasizes prepaid group practice.
64. Richard D. Lyons, "Hot Political Battle Over Health Plan," *New York Times*, September 27, 1970, Section 4, page 9.
65. George G. Reader, "Health Care and Poverty: What Are the Dimensions of the Problem from the Clinician's Point of View?" *Bulletin of the New York Academy of Medicine*, 42 (December, 1966), pp. 1126-1131.
66. "Witness for Medicaid," in *Costs and Delivery of Health Services to Older Americans*, Part 2, p. 520.
67. *Annals of the American Academy of Political and Social Science*, 273 (1951), p. 2.

CHAPTER 7

THE ETHICS OF THE PHYSICIAN IN HUMAN REPRODUCTION

Howard C. Taylor

> The conceptions of life and the world which we call "philosophical" are a product of two factors: one, inherited and religious conception; the other, the sort of investigation which may be called "scientific" using the word in its broadest sense.
>
> —Bertrand Russell

Medical ethics depend on a few essential principles so clearly inherent in the doctor-patient relationship that they continue or recur in each new form of society. These principles include the priority of the patient's welfare, confidentiality of information, avoidance of abusing the medical privilege, loyalty to teacher and colleagues, and the duty to instruct. These fundamentals, however, have always been interpreted in the light of current theological and social values, and these are subject to constant change. Never before, perhaps, have such changes been so rapid as in our own era and in no field have they been so profound as in that emcompassing sexual morality and reproduction. Against this background, and on these shifting foundations, the physician of today must redevelop his code of ethics and outline his area of responsibility.

Sources of Medical Ethics in the Field of Reproduction

In a simpler age medical ethics was—or at least appears to us—largely derived from the profession's own thinking about the physician's relation to his patient and to his colleagues. These principles were embodied in the time-honored Hippocratic Oath, formulated during the classical period in Greece, and still ritualistically taken by graduating students in universities throughout the world. It is useful to start with these clearly stated fundamentals:

> I will look upon him who shall have taught me this Art even as one of my parents. I will share my substance with him and I will supply his necessities if he be in need. I will regard his offspring even as my own brethren, and I will teach them this Art, if they would learn it, without fee or covenant. I will impart this Art by precept, by lecture and by every mode of teaching, not only to my own sons, but to the sons of him who has taught me, and to disciples bound by covenant and oath, according to the Law of Medicine.
>
> The regimen I adopt shall be for the benefit of my patients according to my ability and judgment, and not for their hurt or for any wrong. I will give no deadly drug to any, though it be asked of me, nor will I counsel such, and especially I will not aid a woman to procure abortion. Whatsoever house I enter, there will I go for the benefit of the sick, refraining from all wrongdoing or corruption, and especially from any act of seduction, of male or female, of bond or free. Whatsoever things I see or hear concerning the life of men, in my attendance on the sick or even apart therefrom, which ought not to be voiced abroad, I will keep silence thereon, counting such things to be as sacred secrets.

The fundamentals of medical ethics as conceived of by the physician himself are all embodied in these simple paragraphs. For 2,500 years they have remained pretty much the same, probably because the very nature of the medical vocation makes them essential.

The physician has not, however, been permitted to write all his own rules. Doctrines of the Christian church, and indeed of most other major religions, have played a large role in regulating the physician's conduct. When a religious organization has a dominant position in society, its precepts tend to become a part of the medical ethics of the time, either directly or through the secular law. When the church commands the loyalty of a part of the community only, the physicians of that faith incorporate its teaching in their professional code. Yet the possibilities for moral conflict remain for both physician and patient. In routine situations the rules of the church and the intrinsic medical codes may be reconciled, but in a rare crisis, with life perhaps at stake, the mandates of the two ideologies may present an agonizing dilemma.

The society in which the physician works may also interpose certain obligations that somewhat modify his total commitment to the welfare of a particular patient. The heart of this problem is the balance of values between "rights of the individual" and "obligations to society."

The New York Times of April 21, 1971 reported that the Soviet Union had adopted its own version of the Hippocratic Oath for physicians, effective with the next graduating class of medical students. The Soviet physician undertakes "to guard and develop the noble traditions of Soviet medicine, to be guided in all actions by the principles of Communist morality, and always to remember the high calling of Soviet physician and my responsibility before the people and the Soviet State." No such explicit commitment to society as opposed to the individual is exacted of the Western physician, but there is widespread evidence of a new pressure on the physician to be socially concerned. Perhaps the good of the society and the individual are nearly always the same, but the physician may at times have to tread cautiously between conflicting claims.

Finally, the law of the land has a major effect, for surely it is generally "unethical" for the physician to commit a crime. In making its laws, the state tends to support part of the basic code of medical ethics, but adds variable quantities of theological precepts and modifies the mixture according to dominant social values of the time. The resulting regulations have, of course, a determining influence on what the physician regards as ethical. The majority of physicians in New York abandoned the time-honored prohibition of abortion almost overnight, as soon as the state's legislators, by the narrowest of margins, authorized the interruption of pregnancy simply on the patient's request and a physician's consent.

"Civil disobedience" is a current fashion, recently become somewhat respectable. To the physician, however, such behavior is not new. Acting on what he believes is best for his patient, he has often challenged or evaded the law. The history of the enforcement of statutes respecting contraception and abortion has been replete with examples of acts of medical dissent. Some of these have been overt, designed to attract public attention, as in the case of the opening of an illegal birth control clinic in New Haven which led eventually to the Supreme Court's declaring the Connecticut law unconstitutional. More often the evasion of the law has been less spectacular; for example, the widespread giving of birth-control advice by physicians to their private patients in the face of restrictive laws, and the stretching of indications for theraputic abortions to include some that threatened the mother's life and health only remotely. There remains, then, a shadowy area in which the "ethical" physician, in obedience to his humanitarian principles, will disobey the law.

Extrinsic Values Affecting Medical Ethics in the Field of Reproduction

In no area of medicine are the ethical rules more complicated by considerations outside the physician's proper field than in cases related to reproduction. Indeed, the question has been posed whether birth control is really a medical matter at all, since sickness is not the primary problem. A practical answer is that most techniques now available require medical intervention. Furthermore, the physician's privileged position as adviser in delicate matters of personal behavior is still nearly unique and seems essential. When the need for birth-control services arose, society had no other worker to turn to, so the physician and his assistants have usually assumed the burden without question.

The physician is not only entering a field somewhat foreign to him, but finds that the field itself is in the midst of revolutionary change. We are in a period of transition when the values that most successful peoples have traditionally placed upon procreation are giving place to the necessities of a modern world faced with the threat of collective overpopulation. The admonition "to be fruitful," the duty to produce sons, the prohibition against contraception and abortion, may once have been derived from a high mortality rate and the necessity to maintain the tribe or nation. These biological requirements, embodied in religious teaching, were readily taken over by the physician and for centuries were a part of a generally accepted code of ethics. Yet now a radical change in social values is occurring with profound effects on religious precepts, public policy and personal behavior. For the physician, adapting to the change has often been particularly difficult, partly because of the profession's long commitment to the older system, partly because, for him, the new ideas are not simply academic (as they may be for the sociologist) or impersonal (as for the legislator) but have immediate practical application to his daily work.

In spite of tradition, the last 50 years have of course witnessed a change in the physician's attitude, evident to some degree throughout the world, although much more advanced in some regions than others. The ideas initiating these changes have not appeared simultaneously, but more or less sequentially, accelerating the alteration of the ethical rules. A brief discussion of these ideas may help to explain current medical views.

The idea that maternal health might, under certain circumstances, be adversely affected by pregnancy brought the physician into the field of contraception. The gradual expansion of this concept over the years eventually made it possible for the liberal-minded but ethical physician to give contraceptive advice, at least in the United States and in many other countries, almost as he chooses.

At first he began to give such advice, perhaps even to undertake surgical sterilization, when the complication of a major organic illness made it possible that another pregnancy would be fatal. Some time later it was decided that the welfare of mother and newborn was benefitted by at least two years between births, and contraception began to be prescribed for purposes of spacing. A next step was taken when some psychologists recommended a period of adjustment after marriage before the first pregnancy, and premarital counseling became fashionable. Now, in the face of the current sexual revolution, information to adolescents is often recommended so that they may be protected from the social, psychological, and possible health hazards of out-of-wedlock teenage pregnancy.

The second revolutionary idea, or group of ideas, centered about the concept of overpopulation which now hangs over the minds of thoughtful people as did an earlier vision of the Last Judgment. As a generally literate person, the physician soon realized the implications of excessive procreation, but came more slowly to the realization that society was expecting him to play a major role in alleviating the situation. To the ethical question of how far the physician might intervene in the reproductive life of his individual patient was being added a social responsibility to contribute to the solution of the collective problem.

The role of the physician in programs aimed at "population control" varies from country to country, according to their stage of development, the organization of their health services, and the particular aspect of the problem dominant at the moment in the eyes of public and government. The simplest and original concern was the food supply and the prediction of mass starvation. This calamity has always seemed remote in America and even in the developing countries improved agriculture seems to have advanced the date of this crisis by several decades. The next set of arguments came from the economists. It was shown that a rapid growth rate resulted in a high proportion of children, who, without being productive themselves, made such large demands for education and other social services that too little money might be left in a national budget for industrialization and other economic development projects. These economic considerations, with their patriotic overtones, have had a powerful influence on government policy in some developing countries, and have affected ideas of medical responsibility through official national family-planning programs. In America economic thinking is more narrowly directed at the apparent relationship between large families, poverty, and the swelling welfare rolls. In consequence, efforts are being made to bring birth control to the estimated five million women who do not have access to health facilities. Work on such projects is consistent with the more social orientation of recent medical graduates. Yet in the United States the ecological reasons appear to be having the greatest emotional at present impact at present, providing a moral mandate for the small family. America in particular, it is said, must limit its population because it is consuming more and polluting more than its rightful share. Two children are enough and zero population growth is the goal. The physician, who in his work must struggle with the traffic and in his play is apt to be an outdoorsman, may be particularly susceptible to these arguments.

The physician's duty to his patient and his collective responsibility to society are usually, but not always, in harmony. Consideration will first be given to the medical ethics governing the physician when he acts purely as a physician. The following points will be discussed: (1) the several persons involved in a decision about contraception or abortion; (2) the indications for the ethical prescription of contraception; and (3) ethical problems arising from particular contraceptive techniques.

With this discussion completed, an attempt will be made to outline the physician's responsibility as an agent of society.

For Whom is the Physician Responsible in Prescribing Contraception?

The physician's decision to give or withhold contraceptive advice or services must follow the weighing of factors quite different from those involved in the diagnosis and treatment of illness. Disease can only be considered undesirable. The value of a pregnancy or potential pregnancy will have pluses and minuses of varying weight in different cases.

The physician may of course avoid all responsibility by taking one of two diametrically opposed, but equally absolute, positions. On the one hand, as a strict Catholic perhaps, he may follow the rule that no contraception and of course no abortion is permissible. On the other hand, as a convinced "liberal" he may hold to the opinion that every person has a right to information about contraception and every pregnant woman has a right to an abortion if she wishes it. Neither system involves a medical judgment.

The Patient:[1] On the other hand, if the physician believes that he should contribute to the decision when questions of contraception arise, he must weigh a multitude of factors. These will obviously include the marital status of the patient, her age, the duration of the union if married, children already born, religious convictions which might result in psychological conflicts and many more. Of perhaps greatest importance, however, is the study of the balance between the present needs and the future health and welfare of the patient.

The long view of the patient's life may produce evidence in favor of or against contraception. The future burden an additional child might impose on the health and happiness of a family of marginal economic status has been used as an indication for contraception, for surgical sterilization, and indeed, in some countries, for abortion. It is out of fashion to look at the more distant future for reasons to advise the individual against continued contraception. Advocates of a lower birth rate have taken heart from statistics showing that if all "unwanted births" were eliminated, population increase would cease and a demographic utopia would be at hand. Birth control campaigns have been led by the slogan "No unwanted children." But when is a child unwanted? Is it an unwanted fetus which the mother must carry, an irksome one-year-old, an obtrusive teenager, a grown child graduating from college, or a treasured son or daughter, giving support and comfort in a parent's old age?

Some years ago a young physician came upon his teacher gazing somewhat reflectively at a newspaper photograph of a pretty young girl whose proud parents were announcing her engagement. "You know," he said, "it was just 20 years ago that I saved her life. She must be just over 19 now." Today less medical thought might have been given, and the proposed abortion quickly and routinely carried out.

Whatever the physician's views about overpopulation, he must give first consideration to the individual patient's own welfare, present and future. In general, the value of a child to parents increases, at least to a point, with its age. The unwanted pregnancy of the moment may yield the indispensable son or daughter of the future, and this it is the duty of the physician to make clear.

The Family: The welfare of the patient's family must also be thought of. The physician must consider the wishes and needs of the husband and of other children, as for example the possible psychological disadvantages inherent in the one-child family. The prescription of simple contraceptives may, in view of current practices, be given almost casually, perhaps with the reminder to the childless newly married woman that the years favorable for reproduction are few. For the more permanent or drastic methods of birth control, surgical sterilization (male or female), and abortion, consultation with the spouse seems morally essential, and in many states or countries it is required by law. Family considerations are of course more important and differently oriented in other countries. The need for a son, or even two, which has an economic and almost religious base in many countries of Asia, has only a shadowy parallel in the West.

The Unborn: It is, however, the question of abortion and the physician's responsibility for the fetus which poses the greatest difficulty in the formulation of a modern system of medical ethics. The prohibition against abortion, the most specific admonition in the Hippocratic code, has been the physician's guide for two and a half millennia. The rules of the Roman Catholic Church, inflexible to this day, have confirmed this code. The great Eastern religions, particularly those preoccupied with the preservation of all life, naturally tend to follow similar rules. Many liberals, from their own hierarchy of values, tend also to place great weight on "the sanctity of life."

Opposing this position are two groups. The first are those most impressed with the population problem, especially the very vocal extremist wing who take the simplistic position that the prevention of any birth, however accomplished, is one to the good. The other is made up of those dedicated to the "rights" of the individual, including the right to decide whether or not to bear a child already conceived.

Over the last decade or two numerous conferences have been held to provide an interchange of ideas between representatives of the two views about abortion. In accordance with the current American rule of fraternal courtesy between ideologically bitter opponents, these conferences have been almost ritualistically friendly. Yet essentially there have been no compromises, nor can any be hoped for between the opposing views in their absolute forms.

During the evening social hour following a day's session of such an abortion conference, this writer was engaged in a pleasant conversation with a Catholic priest and scholar. I inquired about a doctrine that has always fascinated me, the belief once held by some theologians that the soul did not enter the fetus till the 40th day in the male, and—perhaps as evidence of medieval antifeminism—at the 80th day for the female. The priest rejected out of hand the idea of any sex discrimination, but admitted that the doctrine of delayed "animation" had appealed to him. I seized upon this with enthusiasm and suggested that it solved our differences about abortion if performed in the early weeks when there was no soul. The priest, unmoved by my enthusiasm, replied, "But we do not know there is no soul until 40 days, and surely we cannot take this risk." My response was to ask when the Church would know, to which my friend calmly replied, "I suppose never." Perhaps this story illustrates the irreconcilable nature of the division.

For the theologian, then, the issue appears to be when the soul enters the embryo; for the humanist it is when life begins. The question can never be definitively answered, although certain state legislatures seem by implication to have given a legal answer in prescribing the week of pregnancy after which abortion is prohibited. Perhaps it will be necessary to abandon attempts at absolutes and to accept a relativistic view that life is gradually acquired, that humanity is not an all-or-none entity but an essence that quantitatively increases as biological development proceeds. Such a concept is probably theologically offensive, and certainly intellectually difficult. It may, however, be the only solution of the present impasse, and a base for the development of a medical ethic that is practical in a modern world and still dedicated to the preservation of human life.

Indeed, there is plentiful evidence that such an ethic is in the process of development. Let us examine the attitude of at least a part of the medical profession toward the interruption of pregnancy, i.e. the destruction of fetal life, at various stages. (a) The suppression of ovulation by means of the oral steriods is, of course, not regarded as an abortion, although as a contraceptive measure it may not be approved. Nevertheless, the attack upon the ovum before fertilization is acceptable to most physicians with a minimum of theological misgiving. (b) Measures which act upon the fertilized ovum, before implantation and before the woman is aware that she has conceived, are subject to somewhat more criticism. Since the intrauterine device presumably acts after conception, it is designated an "abortifacient" and so condemned by such divergent groups as the Catholic clergy and at least certain orthodox Moslems. Yet most non-Catholic physicians are not concerned that they are providing for an abortion, even a biological one, when they insert an intrauterine device. (c) With the delay in the first period, signaling the fact that implantation has occurred, there is admittedly an abrupt change in the point of view of both physician and patient. Nevertheless, an abortion before the 12th week is beginning to be taken lightly, at least in countries that have recognized its legality. (d) As pregnancy progresses, perhaps because there is more of life to be destroyed, the physician becomes more and more hesitant and disturbed in conscience. Many of the laity may not sympathize with this increasing concern, because for them an abortion is an abortion. Unlike the operator, the layman does not have to see the evidence of human form and witness the physiological efforts of the aborted 16-20-week fetus to survive. (e) After a few more weeks of pregnancy, the gradual increase in the humanity of the developing fetus suddenly gives it the right to survive. If it makes 28 weeks, it is "viable," endowed with full legal protection. In a sense, the law in New York State has simply substituted a new absolute, that of 24 weeks, for the old one, the union of two cells at the time of fertilization.

Although some sort of guidelines, theologically or legally sponsored, may have for practical purposes to be sharply defined, it is evident that the physician, at least subconsciously, is ascribing different values to the embryo of different ages. Perhaps with social trends what they are today, it is essential that the physician accept such a quantitative concept if he is to retain his classic dedication to the preservation of life. An abortion at eight weeks might be done "on demand," at 20 weeks only with the most pressing indications.

Society. At this point we will not discuss the physician's general responsibility for the solution of the population problem; this will be referred to later. We ask simply how far the doctor, in dealing with his individual patient, may allow the welfare of society to enter into a decision. Here the physician must tread with the greatest caution, for he may face a conflict of interests.

The need to reduce the birth rate is a real one, but it is not proper for the physician to exploit his privileged position by mounting his own campaign with his personal patients. Perhaps after three children, more justifiably after four or more, the physician may suggest birth control for the patient's own health and economic welfare. The question of whether some parents "should" have more children than others may also intrude itself on the physician's mind and subconsciously color his judgment in some cases. This issue divides itself into two obvious questions: "Should some people have fewer (or no) children?" and "Should some have more?"

There is evidence of a consensus, both medical and public, that some persons should not have children. Certain longstanding state laws providing for the sterilization of the feeble-minded before release from institutions are extreme examples. Beyond such rather obvious reasons for preventing conception, there are some less defensible situations in which the physician will be influenced to varying degrees by the social consequences of procreation. He may consider the likelihood of genetic deficiency, but also the social burdens of out-of-wedlock pregnancy, unemployability, and other characteristics making responsible parenthood less than probable. The physician, as a physician, should relate these indications to his patient's own welfare. In many such cases, some degree of persuasion may be justified by the relative lack of contraceptive services available to underprivileged people in the past.

The opposite idea, that some people "should" have more children, may also occur to some physicians. Some decades ago, there was handwringing over statistics which seemed to show that college graduates were not reproducing themselves. Partly because of the discovery of the population explosion, partly because of the philosophical and political domination of the egalitarian dogma, all ideas of "eugenics" are now in eclipse. Yet it seems probable that intellectual as well as physical competence is to some degree inherited, and it is nearly certain that the home environment, particularly in the first years of life, is a major factor in the individual's future development. The physician may hesitate to give advice that will too drastically curtail the offspring of people with apparently exceptional genetic and cultural qualities. Nothing is certain, but the physician in his counseling may decide to "play the odds" and tell some parents that the children they might have would probably be social assets.

When May Contraceptive Advice be Given by an Ethical Physician?

By the expansion of the health indication, as has been shown, the occasions on which contraception may be prescribed by the ethical physician have greatly multiplied. There are still differences over what technique of birth control is permissible; for example, many disapprove of surgical sterilization for the very young or the childless. There are also other questions: When may a physician give a prescription if requested, and when should he initiate the subject and actively urge the practice of contraception? Finally, there are still a few uncertain situations in which advice and services should perhaps be refused.

In the presence of organic disease, which would make a pregnancy hazardous to life, the physician's clear duty is to provide the most efficient and acceptable means to prevent another conception. Perhaps a similar case, in which the physician has a clear duty, is the condition called "grand multiparity," the history of a considerable number of children already born, imposing upon the mother the physical burden for their care and the statistically proven increasing hazard of each succeeding pregnancy.

Many obstetricians consider the "spacing" of pregnancy so important that they regard the routine offering of contraceptive advice after each pregnancy as a responsibility of the physician. Such advice is especially necessary in Western countries, where decline in breast feeding has removed a useful, if undependable, physiological bar to an early recurrence of pregnancy. In the undeveloped countries, spacing is important for the opposite reason: Here, if a new pregnancy occurs in spite of lactation, the milk supply will be reduced and, in the absence of materials for artificial feeding, the first child will suffer from various forms of malnutrition. One of these, kwashiorkor, is a frequent affliction of "the last child but one" in some tropical countries. The practice of routinely giving birth control advice after the first pregnancy surely seems consistent with current views of medical responsibility.

Women approaching marriage are often advised to consult a gynecologist for the detection of the rather rare, but still possible, anatomical defects that might provide difficulties in coitus, conception, or pregnancy. These premarital sessions provide an opportunity to answer questions about the physical aspects of marriage, and usually include advice on contraception. Few American physicians today would regard this practice as unethical, but it was still debated not so many years ago, and in some countries the giving of contraceptive advice to childless women is still legally forbidden.

The revolution in sexual mores, and the direct availability of contraceptive devices through other than medical channels, has perhaps made any refusal of a physician to prescribe a little ridiculous. Nevertheless, an ethical problem still exists with respect to contraceptive advice or prescription to those who are unmarried and not about to be married. Here rules have not been set and a great diversity in the practice of physicians varies widely, perhaps partly because this situation presents itself in so many different settings. At one extreme, there is the mature woman, perhaps already divorced, who merely wants advice on some technique of contraception other than the one she is already practicing. Less clear is the proper response to the college student, involved in a serious but probably temporary relationship and already running the risk of pregnancy. Many physicians, recognizing the frequency of premarital intercourse or perhaps even approving, will supply the needed information. But, at what age is he ethically justified in doing this? At 21, at 18, at 16, at 14? When must the parents' consent be obtained?

The physician must also consider whether he may have an actual responsibility to provide contraceptive services to the unmarried girl who has already had one out-of-wedlock pregnancy. Repetitions of such pregnancies are known to be common. If the physician supplies contraceptive advice he may further encourage promiscuity; if he does not, he invites another out-of-wedlock pregnancy. Most physicians will surely feel that one illegitimate child is sufficient justification for contraception, but the ethical principles involved are complicated. The conscientious physician must certainly do all that his time and energies will permit to prevent these repetitions. Unfortunately, such service is time-consuming, and the women who are particularly prone to repeated out-of-wedlock pregnancies are not well supplied with medical care or social guidance.

Ethical Considerations with Respect to Particular Contraceptive Techniques

Beside the ethical aspects of contraception in general, there are particular characteristics of various techniques which the conscientious physician must weigh. The three most important are the health hazard, the relative permanency of the infertility produced, and—in some cases—special theological or moral implications.

Although birth control cannot be regarded as a hazardous practice by the usual standards of medical therapy, there is a minute risk associated with certain methods. These risks are not statistically demonstrable except when large numbers of cases are analyzed, but deaths have certainly occurred in association with the steroid oral contraceptives and the I.U.D., as well as in surgery for abortion or sterilization. The benefits to be derived from these measures must be balanced against the possibility of accidents. In general these are so infrequent that both physician and patient may tend largely to disregard them.

With respect to the health hazard, the question is nevertheless often raised whether the prospective user must be fully apprised of the risk involved. This situation is indeed only a special example of the broader question facing the medical profession today, that of "informed consent" by the patient before any significant medical procedures. The resolution of the problem, with its medico-legal as well as ethical undertones, is not simple. The mere introduction of the idea of danger may immediately induce psychological reactions unfavorable to the success of the therapy. Few people can regard themselves as subject to average statistical chances, and the statistically correct information that there is one chance in 30 thousand of a fatal accident with the pill may well result in a quite erroneous subjective appreciation of the chances.

Misgivings are also occasionally expressed about supplying pills as part of certain programs of assistance to developing countries. This issue is usually resolved by noting that millions of American women are themselves using the pill, and by providing responsible officials of the countries concerned with all available scientific reports on the health hazards. To some critics these are still not sufficient justifications, and it has been suggested that packages of pills destined for the women of a developing country should carry a health warning, like cigarettes in America. The futility of the effort to achieve individual, fully informed consent becomes apparent, however, when it is remembered that the majority of women in many of these countries cannot read.

The responsibility assumed by the physician will also vary greatly in relation to the permanence of the procedure recommended. The so-called "reversible" methods may be almost routinely prescribed in some societies. The operations for the sterilization of male or female must be preceded by a careful survey of the patient's present situation and future needs as far as predictable.

The final category, and for many the most important, is that of the theological implications. Medical ethics must be deeply concerned with these values if either physician or patient is committed to them. The pertinent religious and moral principles have been derived from two sources. One is the almost timeless apprehension about sex in general, but particularly about sex when not for the purpose of procreation. St. Thomas Aquinas wrote, "In so far as the generation of offspring is impeded, it is a vice against nature which happens in every carnal act from which generation cannot follow," and this view has been central to the Roman Catholic position even since the 13th century. Such opinions, though less explicitly expressed and adhered to, have been shared by many

Protestant thinkers. The second principle, supported by most religions as well as by a secular humanistic philosophy, is the absolute "sanctity of human life." The individual birth-control techniques must be evaluated on the basis of these two concepts.

Periodic abstinence, or the "safe-period" method, is generally approved for Roman Catholics, with the reservation that marriage should not be entered into with the intent never to have children and that pregnancy should be avoided by the "safe-period" method only when there is a special need. Although sometimes irreverently termed "Vatican roulette," the safe period can be highly effective, if practiced according to strict rules by intelligent and highly motivated people.

The principle of the safe period depends on the observed facts that ovulation, in women of regular 28-day periods, occurs on or about the 15th day of the cycle, that the ovum is then capable of fertilization for not more than 24 hours, and that sperm can retain their fertilizing capacity for not over three days. Possible variations in the exact day of ovulation require abstinence for from 5 to 8 days each month for women with regular cycles and any tendency to irregularity in cycle length makes a longer interval necessary. Nevertheless, the safe period is effective for couples willing to exercise this degree of restraint, and no voice seems now to be raised against use of this "natural method" by married people.

The "traditional" or obstructive methods. A number of methods, some time-honored, others based on a somewhat modern technology, work by preventing the sperm from reaching the ovum in the uterus or Fallopian tube. The methods include coitus interruptus, the obstructive devices worn in the vagina or over the cervix, certain spermacidal preparations for placement in the vagina and the male sheath or condom. All have the advantage of being fairly reliable temporary measures with no proven deleterious physiologic or pathologic consequences. All are forbidden by the Church, again for reasons epitomized in another often-quoted statement in the *Summa Theologica* of Aquinas:

> The inordinate emission of semen is against the good of nature, which is the conservation of the species; hence, after the sin of homicide, by which human nature actually existing is destroyed, this kind of sin, by which the generation of human nature is impeded, seems to hold second place.

Perhaps these methods, except possibly for the vaginal diaphragm, have become rather irrelevant to medical ethics in the United States, since all are readily available to the informed laity and medical intervention is scarcely needed.

Pharmacologic contraception—"the pill." A new era in the history of birth control began with the discovery that substances identical with or chemically related to the natural steroid hormones of the ovary and testis would prevent ovulation and so provide security against pregnancy. The method is highly dependable, steadily decreasing in cost to the user, and relatively free from immediate side effects. The occurrence of serious complications in a minute fraction of the users tends to be brushed aside, partly on the statistical evidence that the prevented pregnancies would have produced substantially more health difficulties.

This method of birth control is based on a hitherto unavailable mechanism. No obstruction is offered at the time of intercourse to the union of sperm and ovum, and indeed no contraceptive act occurs before or during intercourse. There is simply no ovum available during the cycle when the medication is being taken. High hopes existed that the method would receive Papal approval, but, consistent with the Church's traditional position, this approval was not given. This decision may have had little effect in the United States where statistics show that a high percentage of Catholics do use contraception, but in certain countries, notably in Latin America, the program for slowing the rate of population increase received a serious setback.

A possible future development of the pharmacological approach to contraception offers another interesting, and to some amusing, theological problem. The rather frivolously designated "morning-after" pill is composed of chemical substances similar in nature to those used in the common suppressor of ovulation, but in higher dosage. Although statistical proof of effectiveness is for obvious reasons difficult to obtain, it appears probable that during the first few days after intercourse the ovum may be destroyed during its passage through the Fallopian tube. Since the ovum has possibly now been fertilized, the "morning-after" pill may have to be characterized as an abortifacient, in a strict biological and theological sense.

The intrauterine device. The history of the intrauterine contraceptive device (the I.U.D.) is particularly illustrative of the transitory nature of specific items in the code of medical ethics. As the Gräfenberg Ring, it was denounced to all medical students during the 1920's and 30's as immoral and, perhaps worse, as an inevitable source of infection. Reintroduced to Western medicine in somewhat different form in 1959, it was soon widely accepted and has become one of the techniques on which many programs of population control have depended. Since after the initial insertion little further thought need be given by the user, the method has proved especially applicable in developing countries where the schedule of pill-taking may be difficult to remember and home conditions are not conducive to the continued use of the traditional methods. The intrauterine device is highly reliable, but not completely, since about three pregnancies occur per year among each 100 users. Some usually minor complaints are fairly common, but serious or fatal complications have rarely been reported.

Yet the intrauterine device poses special theologically based ethical problems for some physicians and patients. The biological mechanisms by which it produces this relative infertility have not yet been absolutely demonstrated. Accumulating evidence tends to show, however, that the I.U.D. creates an unfavorable environment in the uterine cavity so that the fertilized ovum is either destroyed or is lost because it cannot implant. Had the action been to block spermatozoa in their ascent or even to cause a precipitate discharge of the unfertilized ovum, as was once claimed, this method, as contraception, would be thought bad enough. The postconceptional destruction of the fertilized ovum can, however, also be interpreted as abortion and as such it has been condemned.

The "abortion" from the I.U.D., if this is indeed the mechanism of its action, occurs before the date of the expected period, so that the woman is not aware of a pregnancy nor has she made any conscious attempt to terminate a particular pregnancy. The majority of American physicians who insert the I.U.D. are, like their patients, apparently unconcerned with the fine question of whether a life has begun. The use of the I.U.D. is certainly considered by some Catholic physicians as a more serious step than use of the pill. Nor is this view restricted to Catholic doctrine, a point strongly brought home to me recently when I attended a lecture given in Djakarta by an Indonesian professor of obstetrics and gynecology. As an orthodox Moslem, he condemned the I.U.D. as an abortifacient and quoted as his principal authority the work of a deceased Protestant professor of obstetrics and gynecology at the University of Göttingen!

Surgical sterilization. Surgical sterilization for either the male or the female is being increasingly resorted to as an almost perfectly reliable method which frees the individual from all future concerns with calendars, pills or gadgets. In sophisticated societies it is a convenience; in the less educated or motivated it provides security against the discontinuance which so often occurs among "acceptors" of the I.U.D. or the pill.

The theological objections to surgical sterilization are the same as those for other forms of contraception. It appears to outside observers, however, that the initial sin, once committed and repented of, can be forgiven, and the operation can thus be less onerous than repeated resort to temporary contraception. Certainly in at least one Catholic country, Puerto Rico, female sterilization has been a very common practice.

The special responsibility of the physicien in advising or performing sterilization stems from its relative permanence. Before advising or undertaking surgical sterilization he must therefore consider whether the married couple are really convinced that they want no more children, or even whether their marriage is stable, for should it be dissolved either partner might be handicapped in the search for another union by his or her artificially produced sterility.

In some of the developing countries—in certain states in India, for example—some doubts have been expressed about the ethical justification for providing "incentives" and "quotas" for sterilization procedures. Some programs have set quotas for the number of such operations to be performed per year per clinic, and small payments are provided for the man who submits to the operation as well as to the "referrer" who brings him to the clinic. Although the population problem in India seems to justify such a program, there are critics who disapprove of this system of incentives as "coercive."

Abortion. On account of the second life involved, abortion has traditionally and properly been regarded as the most radical method of birth control. To the more pragmatically minded, it might perhaps rank second to surgical sterilization because the latter is usually permanent.

We have discussed the theological considerations that affect the attitude of the physician. For centuries these provided a secure base for medical behavior. Now, however, the pressure exerted by social considerations and the ever-widening doctrine of "individual right" have drastically altered the law in many countries and states. Except that in predominantly Catholic countries abortion is not generally countenanced, the liberalization of the law seems not to have followed any particular cultural or political pattern. Thus we find abortion available, with few restrictions, in such divergent societies as Japan, Russia and the Communist countries of East Europe, Britain, New York State, and Hawaii. The most liberal of all laws was that approved in New York in 1970, which allows abortion up to the 24th week of pregnancy on the request of the patient and the consent of a physician. The lack of any residency requirement has given New York the title of "abortion capital of the world," and has encouraged the development of highly profitable "abortion clinics" available to patients from other parts of the country through an organized referral system.

Over the last few years, several systems of medical ethics have evolved, relating to different legal regulations for the performance of abortion. As one travels from country to country, even from state to state in America, one finds the physician facing different, and often distressing, dilemmas.

Where abortion is categorically forbidden or the permissible indications are few and precise, the illegal abortionist flourishes with a consequent higher mortality and morbidity. The woman who is determined to have an abortion often first consults her personal physician. He is then faced by the humane, if not ethical, decision of whether to refer her to a "good abortionist" or to wash his hands of the affair, as the law requires, thus perhaps allowing her to fall into the hands of a dangerous amateur or unscrupulous criminal. The prevalence of illegal abortion in some countries has had the paradoxical effect of diminishing the opposition to contraception (even, it is said, that of the Church) in order to lessen the greater evil.

In the middle range of legal liberality, "therapeutic" abortion may be permitted to preserve "the life or health of the mother." Until recently, laws of this kind were the basis for medical action throughout the United States and still probably prevail over most of the world. The vagueness about "the life or the health of the mother" has left room for varied interpretations by individual physicians and groups of physicians. A degree of hypocrisy often provided the needed indication, if the patient were in a position to seek and find a sufficiently liberal or compliant physician. Certainly the well-to-do, who of course were able to obtain more medical care of all all kinds, were more often able to have borderline "therapeutic" abortions.

When the law is fully liberalized, as in New York State, to permit "abortion on demand," the rules are all changed and the burden of obligation reversed. Mechanisms to prevent or limit the performance of abortions are replaced by the responsibility to provide services. Many physicians were understandably confused when thus required to change the attitudes of a lifetime as a result of a bill passed almost capriciously by a majority of one in the New York State legislature.

The weight of these changes has been felt most by specialists and departments of obstetrics and gynecology. The majority of non-Catholic specialists are unemotionally adapting themselves to the new situation, but there are exceptions, one at each extreme. Some few are becoming "abortion specialists"and are regarded with a degree of contempt by their colleagues for their alleged venality. At the other extreme are obstetrician-gynecologists who decline to be involved, risking the criticism of refusing to bear their share of an unpleasant task. The Catholic hospitals understandably do not permit abortions, but the Catholic physician now faces more than ever before the dilemma of whether to refer an apparently deserving case to another physician or clinic for the operation he cannot, or will not, do himself.

The amorphous present state of medical ethics with respect to abortion may be expected to continue for some time. Doctrines elevating the right of the individual, while diminishing ideas of personal responsibility, are in the ascendency. Time and experience will produce some rules, although they will probably not reinstate the old ones. Deeper insights into what is good for the individual and for society will produce future revolutions perhaps as fundamental as the present ones. It may be predicted then that some order will eventually be imposed on the present system, based as it is on conflicting sets of ethical, religious, and social doctrines.

Differences Between the Responsibility of the Profession and the Ethics of the Physician

Some differences between the responsibilities of the medical profession as a whole and the ethical code of the individual physician have already been suggested. It is now necessary to analyze these differences in more detail and to examine the points of conflict.

Society may of course take many actions that an individual may not. The example of violence in warfare is currently the most obvious one, if a bit harsh for use in the present context. Within the medical profession itself, however, there may at times be conflict between the obligations and actions appropriate to the public health administrator at one extreme and the family practitioner at the other. But the collective and individual functions are not sharply segregated into two separate medical professions, and a proportion of each is contained in almost every physician's work. What has been called the "Arrowsmith dilemma," after the hero of Sinclair Lewis' novel, is often present, although perhaps usually unacknowledged.

One conflict in the area of reproductive medicine is between the need of society for reduced population growth and the benefits of children to the particular wife and husband. The child which to some societies is another mouth to feed may also be the family's chief future source of security, material and psychological. An attempt has been made to resolve the difficulty through terminology; "family planning" may be acceptable where "population control" is barred. Whether voluntary "family planning" can be the means to achieve an ultimate stable world population is doubted by many demographers. For the moment, however, the concept is helpful to the physician's conscience.

It appears, then, that the medical profession does have to recognize two separate and occasionally conflicting obligations. Acting as a member of the profession, and speaking publicly as an individual, the physician has a major opportunity and equal responsibility to help solve overpopulation. When, however, he is dealing with an individual woman or man who has accepted him as principal confidante and adviser, it is this particular patient's welfare that must come first.

The Responsibility of the Profession in Family Planning

The social aspects of medicine have received increasing attention in recent years, and the profession has been under criticism for its alleged neglect of community responsibilities. Such criticism has come from many sources, ranging from high government officials with constituencies that must be satisfied to undergraduate medical students who disapprove of their elders. Lower standards of health care in the city ghettos and among the rural poor are laid at the door of the profession, which is expected somehow to provide a remedy; although the situation, in some form, is prevalent the world over and in many so-called developing regions the disproportionate concentration of physicians in the cities, at the expense of the countryside, is even greater than in Europe and the United States.

The proud traditions of medicine still seem to lay a particular duty upon the individual physician to make personal sacrifices beyond those required of men in other callings. Perhaps physicians also have a moral responsibility to move voluntarily into the areas of greatest need. As in the past, some few physicians will heed this call. The contribution of most physicians, certainly those already established, will not require such drastic steps. They may return to an older custom and decide to volunteer more time in wards and clinics. Their greatest assistance may come, however, from the influence they can bring to bear on taxpayers and budget officers to give increased financial support for health services, and on their own professional societies to revise their policies for the changing conditions of today.

Among the physician's increasing social responsibilities, the specific ones that are relative to reproduction are important. The responsibilities in this field seem to fall into two large categories:

(a) *The obligation to inform.* The urgency of the population problem is now so great that anyone who may be influential should help disseminate information about it. The physician may play a special role, for he is credited with some special knowledge of the subject and is apt to be consulted when decisions about birth control are being made. In spite of the many public sources of information available to people in America, the physician's views thus remain important. In the developing countries where communications through the press, the radio and television are limited, the attitudes and pronouncements of the medical profession may be a decisive factor in the success of a particular program.

(b) *The obligation to assure service.* The educated and well-to-do married couples in the United States almost all use some technique of family planning, and have done so for years. On the other hand, there are still an estimated five million underprivileged women who do not have ready access to family planning services. Less publicized statistical evidence from the records of maternity hospitals shows that therapeutic abortions as well as surgical sterilizations are much more commonly performed for private than for ward patients. The service rendered may then actually be inversely related to the needs.

This maldistribution of contraceptive attention can cynically be ascribed to our medical fee-for-service system and to an extent this is at least indirectly involved. The ignorance of the patient about what is actually available to her is often a more important consideration. Instruction in birth-control techniques requires time, a priceless commodity in a doctor's day. Formerly, when the care of the indigent depended largely on service volunteered by the physician, the profession could be blamed entirely for not giving it adequately. With the substitution of a system of remuneration for city hospital and clinic work, inadequate services must be blamed on insufficient staff, itself dependent on small budgets and so ultimately on the tax payer. Nevertheless, the physician still has a responsibility to assure adequate contraceptive and, in some states, abortion services for the underprivileged who desire them, either by his own greater efforts or through pressures he can bring on government. If he fails he must give up his support of our present system of delivering medical services, and back some alternative organization that might be more successful.

The ethical obligation to provide information and service in family planning rests particularly heavily on the obstetrician and on the public health physician concerned with maternal and child health. For there are many reasons for believing that the expansion of maternity services and the inclusion in this service of family planning sessions may be the best way to convey information on this topic to the masses of uninformed persons.

The concentration of attention on the woman who is pregnant or has recently been delivered offers many advantages. Services to women at these times are directed toward that part of the population most susceptible to pregnancy, young women who have recently demonstrated their fertility. Such a person recognizes the subject of birth control, at least for the purpose of child-spacing, as an acceptable topic for discussion. The attendants, doctors or midwives, to whom the woman has confided her own safety will also be trusted in such matters as family planning. Its association with health services to mother and child will place family planning in a context most acceptable to the people, and—where this may be important—to church and state.

The continued increase in population will eventually make universal limitation of family size essential. The medical profession, especially the part concerned with maternal and child health, has a particular opportunity and therefore responsibility. The organizational responsibility requires that no woman be discharged from a maternity hospital without the opportunity to learn the means of child-spacing. In the many parts of the world where women are still delivered in their homes without trained assistance, it is the duty of the profession to exert political pressure on their governments to expand the health services, especially in the rural areas, to make family planning possible.

The Ethics of the Physician

The responsibilities of the physician are directed to the same ultimate objectives as those of the profession, but the discharge of his duties is subject to somewhat difficult rules. The profession may be collectively devoted to the goal of population control and so may strongly support the opening of family planning clinics and the extension of maternity services as a base for a more systematic birth control coverage. The physician may not make his personal contribution to the solution of the population problem by the exercise of undue persuasion upon his individual patient.

With this as an example of how medical ethics may differ from the responsibility of the profession, we may conclude by trying to list what appear to be the essentials of a current code for the physician himself.

1. The absolute priority of the individual patient's welfare must remain the cornerstone of the physician's system of ethics. "The regimen I adopt shall be for the benefit of my patients according to my ability and judgement" remains as valid as when this part of the oath was first conceived.

What is for the benefit of the patient, particularly where medicine is concerned with reproduction, may be complicated and subject to different conclusions according to the "judgment" of particular physicians. Some, believing in the patient's right to the services will supply contraceptive information, even undertake an abortion, on a simple request. These give up all but the technical functions of the physician. Before prescribing or acting, the more conscientious and "ethical" physician will consider with his patient, not only her present needs but her future welfare, the physical as well as psychological effects of a particular decision, the consequences for her family and perhaps for her church affiliations.

2. Confidentiality is a part of the old code and is particularly relevant in a medical field concerned with sex and reproduction. The changing status of the parent-child and husband-wife relationship raises a few new questions. The physician may listen sympathetically to the 16-year-old's story of her sex problems, but will he prescribe contraceptives without discussion with a parent? He may receive in confidence the wife's confession of an out-of-wedlock pregnancy, but should he be an accomplice to the wife's deception by undertaking and concealing an abortion? The physician should refuse acts that are clandestine or deceptive, but the confidentiality of the information received must remain inviolate.

3. The patient's ability to make a truly voluntary decision may be compromised in many ways. She may come to her physician with her mind made up as a result of chance contacts with one of several attitudes prevalent today. Here the physician's duty may be to present some points for the opposing view, so that decisions may be made on the basis of at least partially balanced judgment. A more serious breach of professional ethics occurs when the physician uses his privileged position to impose his own views, especially those derived from nonmedical value systems. The conservative physician who is guided by traditional theological doctrines may explain these to his patient, but may not usurp the role of the clergy in trying to enforce the rules derived from such doctrines. More common today, and perhaps even more to be condemned, is the case of the physician who is himself

seriously convinced of the urgency of the population problem and uses his consulting room to impose some current idea such as "zero population growth" or the moral duty to have no more than two children.

Family planning as now conceived of supposes a voluntary limitation by the parents of the number of their children. But what is voluntary? What is coercive? The transition from one to the other is not sharp; indeed, there is a spectrum of situations with varying proportions of each quality. The step away from a truly voluntary approach begins simply with the presentation of a one-sided point of view. Thereafter the spectrum of intensified persuasion proceeds through slanted education, propaganda, perhaps "brainwashing." Economic sanctions against large families and rewards for small families, which are under discussion, have a different kind of coercive element. These perhaps should not be found too abhorrent, since they have long existed in an unplanned form. Poverty for both generations is often the penalty of much childbearing.

The world situation is rapidly changing. As the time of the ultimate catastrophe from the "population explosion" approaches—and in some parts of the world this may be very near—some forms of coercion or incentive for people not to reproduce will be decreed by society. In that day, the physician's primary allegiance will change too. In the meantime, when he is functioning in his role as physician, he must put his patient's personal welfare first and lead her to a decision as nearly voluntary as circumstances will permit.

4. The physician, with religious convictions, whether he be a Catholic opposed to all forms of contraception or a Protestant opposed at least to abortion, cannot and must not be expected to give advice or services contrary to the dictates of conscience. Is such a physician then obligated to explain to his patient where such services may be obtained? Fortunately the laity in the United

States usually understands these relationships and this dilemma need rarely be faced.

5. The law of the land is certainly a part of the ethical code of the physician. Under two circumstances, in the area of reproductive medicine, it may be broken by the ethical physician. One is where an old law, such as that existing in Connecticut until a few years ago forbidding even the practice of contraception, has become generally disregarded, and unenforceable. The other is when some law is so repugnant to a physician that he is willing to flaunt it publicly and take the consequences of his civil disobedience. Breaking the law clandestinely robs the act of most of its virtue and as a rule makes it medically unethical.

6. The welfare of the individual and the good of society are sometimes in conflict. Fortunately, the claims of each are usually parallel: Neither an illegitimate child nor a genetically defective one is usually an asset to parents or community. The physician today should expand his social commitments, but when he is acting as a physician he must place his responsibility to his personal patient first. His social responsibilities are chiefly to ensure that the people are informed so that they may make intelligent decisions and that clinics or other services are available to which they may go if they wish.

This chapter is an attempt to formulate the principles which should currently govern medical ethics and the profession's responsibilities with respect to the problems of human reproduction. Perhaps the attempt has resulted in a list that is too precise. Many will disagree and wish to add, to subtract or certainly to change the emphasis. Any formulation must be vulnerable, partly because of present conflicts in goals and values, partly because changes in both are ceaselessly taking place.

The physician himself is faced with the contradictions between his own code, giving top priority to the welfare of his patient, the traditional commands and prohibitions of his own religious views and the evolving systems of secular, socially derived values. Since a conflict of loyalty may be agonizingly difficult, some physicians adhere tenaciously to the old, others rush almost hysterically after the new. Through this maze of contradictory influences the thoughtful physician must find his own course with compassion, but with cool and informed judgement.

Note

1. Throughout this chapter the candidate for birth control advice or service is designated as a "patient," for although sickness is usually not involved, there is no satisfactory alternative term for the physician's clients. The patient is designated as "she," partly because more than half of the burden is the woman's, partly because for the writer, as for every obstetrician-gynecologist, all patients are feminine.

CHAPTER 8

BIRTH DEFECTS

THE ETHICAL PROBLEM

Leroy Augenstein

In our society many people have the opinion that once a child is conceived, it has the right not to be aborted. And once this child is born, it acquires all kinds of rights and privileges that are guaranteed by our laws. An unconceived individual, however, is a hypothetical thing. It has no rights. Thus, we need to ask: Should an unconceived individual have any rights? In particular, should some unconceived individuals have the right never to be conceived at all?

In deciding that a child should have the right not to be conceived, one must ask what that child might have accomplished had it been conceived. Let us examine briefly three specific kinds of congenital abnormalities that research indicates are genetically controlled.

The first of these is anencephaly, which means, literally, "no brain." Such a child is born with only the primitive brain stem, but none of the higher brain functions intact. Fortunately, and I think I use the term advisably, these individuals do not survive very long. Those who do are literally vegetables.

A second related malformation is hydrocephaly, in which there is an abnormal accumulation of fluid in the ventricles of the brain. Unless this is diagnosed almost immediately after birth, and a tricky operation is performed to put in a drain, the hydrocephalic child will have an I.Q. of 25 or less.

The third of this unholy trio is spina bifida. With this defect, the vertebrae do not close completely to form a protective arch above the spinal cord. However, in many cases, a good surgeon can take a piece of bone from the leg and fuse the vertebrae so that the individual can have a fairly normal life.

If a set of parents has one child with any of these abnormalities, the chance that the next live birth will be a similar one is somewhat in the neighborhood of 5 per cent. However, the probability that the next pregnancy will be another such child or a still-born or a miscarriage is one in four.

Mongolism is another malady where the probabilities are known quite accurately. Mongoloids have an extra chromosome—47 instead of the normal 46. Even though the extra one is one of the tiniest of human chromosomes, it really "messes up the works." In some cases this extra chromosome becomes stuck to one of the others and "goes piggy back." If this happens in the egg, the chance of another such child at the next conception is one in three. However, in some cases the extra chromosome comes along "free for the ride," so to speak. The probability for this is determined almost exclusively by the age of the mother. Often these children are called "children of a tired womb." For a mother 20 years old, the chances of having a mongoloid child are about two in 10 thousand; by the time the mother is 30, the chances are close to one in one thousand, at age 40, they are one in 100; and by the time the mother is 45 to 49, the chances may be one in 40 to one in 25.

To emphasize the moral dilemma, let me refer to two letters I received recently. The first was from a couple who have five children. Their three oldest are normal young people; a daughter of 20, a boy of 18, and another boy of 15. Five years ago they had twins with the following defects: both were born with microcephaly (their heads were very small and were deficient in a number of the vital mental functions); both were born blind and had epileptic seizures; one of them was born deaf; and the other had a very rare blood disorder. Further, one of them screamed 16 to 18 hours a day so that at the age of five years the child weighed only 17 pounds from lack of food.

The mother asked in her letter, "My daughter is just now becoming engaged. If she marries and has children, what are the chances that her children will have these defects?"

The second letter was from a young high-school senior, very much in love and hoping to get married when she graduates. She has spina bifida and was also concerned about her chances of transmitting this defect to her future children.

Both letters concluded, "Any help you can give . . . will be very much appreciated."

Let us discuss what it means to give these people help. Science alone cannot do the job; science can only supply the knowledge and the tools.

From the diagnosis of the young lady who wrote the second letter, it was obvious that she had received from both parents a defective gene of a particular kind known as a recessive trait. Thus, she will pass on one defective gene to any child she will have. Whether her children will exhibit this trait or not will depend exclusively upon the father. If he has two good genes for this trait, all their children will receive one good gene and one bad gene.

Accordingly, they would not have spina bifida but would carry one recessive gene for this trait. However, if the father happened to have one good gene and one bad one, the chances for the defect would be 50-50 at each conception. If, in fact, she married a man with spina bifida (even if, like her, he had had it corrected), then we would immediately know that both of them would pass on a defective gene, so that the probability that their children would have either spina bifida or something worse would be 100 per cent.

In fact, this young lady was lucky. Her two defective genes made it almost certain that her central nervous system would not develop properly while she was still in her mother's womb. She could have been born with anencephaly or hydrocephaly, the other two related birth defects mentioned above.

A second kind of help for this young lady that may come from science is that in the future we may be able to correct defective genes chemically. It is scientific fact that the heredity of all cells is determined by their nucleic acid (DNA), and that the heredity of bacteria can be manipulated. We can take bacteria with one kind of obvious properties, grind them up, extract the hereditary chemical DNA,and put it into a second kind of bacteria, with the result that some of the latter bacteria are transformed so that they take on the properties of the first group. We have not been able to do this in human beings in a controlled way; however, all of us, throughout our lives, have had many of our cells transformed by viruses that are nothing more than "packaged DNA." Viruses consist of DNA with a protein wrapped around the outside for protection. When such a virus comes up to a cell, it will attach itself, tail first, and dissolve a hole in the cell wall, after which the DNA is injected inside.

Usually the transformation caused by the viruses is an adverse one, because we get a snuffly nose, or a fever blister, or polio, or even leukemia.

If we can figure out how DNA exerts its control, then in theory at least we can make made-to-order changes in a human being. It seems almost certain that some workable technique will be found for manipulating human heredity, thereby opening up fantastic new vistas of preventive medicine. However, in many cases we can't wait for the adult to request such treatment. If a child is born with anencephaly, it is too late; we can't make a new brain. The worst abnormalities should be corrected prior to conception.

Since there are anywhere from 10^8 to 10^9 sperms given off at an ejaculation, the chances of getting the necessary corrections into all of them is quite small. The place where we would probably go if we were to use this method is into the ovaries. At puberty the female has all 100 thousand of her eggs formed. This is her lifetime supply, and she will ovulate only 500 to one thousand of them before she dies. So if we could get the necessary corrections into this relatively small number of cells, then theoretically we could prevent the occurrence of at least some of the abnormalities.

Knowledge of predictable birth defects and heredity manipulation applies to situations such as that presented in the second letter, but not necessarily in the first, which described an unusually complex situation. Normally twins' defects do not go together as a package, so that I anticipated that there had been other problems in the pregnancy. I learned that the mother had hemorrhaged rather severely during the second and third months of pregnancy, just when the central nervous system is being formed. Possibly this caused the multiple defects. However, the mother had also hemorrhaged badly during one of her earlier pregnancies. Thus, we aren't sure what to tell her daughter, and, in this case, are unable to predict accurately because the hemorrhaging might have been controlled genetically.

There is, however, another kind of service that we may be able to give this young lady. It is now possible, in monkeys halfway through pregnancy and after all the vital organs are formed, to remove the fetus from the mother's womb, inspect it, and put it back with no obvious ill effects. Some people propose that we develop this technique for human beings. For example, in the case of the first young lady, we expect problems in the fourth or fifth month of pregnancy. Therefore, some argue, if the fetus is removed, and if inspection shows it to be defective, it can be aborted.

So much for science, which supplies the tools and the knowledge. Let us proceed to the ethics. We must now ask, "What would we like man to be?" "Do we desire to change him?"

Let us look ahead to the day when we have developed the technique for fetal inspection. Imagine that you are impaneled on a jury sitting next door to an operating room where an inspection operation is performed in the fourth or fifth month of pregnancy. The doctor announces over the loudspeaker system that he has just inspected the fetus and found that it is destined to have anencephaly. The surgeon now asks a very simple question on which you must vote: Should this child be aborted or put back to go full term? How would you vote?

This is about as black-and-white a case as I can make. Let's make it more difficult. The next operation is performed, and the doctor says over the loudspeaker that this developing child will have PKU. This means that the child cannot handle phenylanine—one of our essential foodstuffs. A child with the two PKU defective genes will end up with an I.Q. of 25 or 30 at the most, unless he is kept on a restrictive diet for at least 10 years and, in many cases, for most of his life. Even if the child is kept on the restrictive diet, the best that can be hoped for is an average I.Q. of 100. Furthermore, it is important to realize how difficult it is to keep the child on such a diet. Even though parents are diligent, the child will be continually at the neighbors begging for a crust of bread or a cookie, and much of the brain damage in these children is the result of softhearted neighbors.

Realizing what will be in store for such a PKU child, would you vote to abort it? Would you vote definitely not to abort it? Would you be willing to sit on a board to draw up a list of defects that would automatically mean abortion? Suppose no one else would serve, would you decide alone?

The real question is: Where does one draw the line? And who draws the line? Decisions about utilizing the new scientific tools will require that scientists, humanists, religious and political leaders, must work closely together.

If you knew that you carried a seriously defective gene, would you want to have it corrected with one of the viruses? More important, do you know that *every* person has an average of five to 10 genes that are so defective that if they are matched up at conception there is a good chance of a real catastrophe?

As we consider the following questions, remember that we are not talking about an unknown stranger but about you and me, your family and my family. Man is different from a rabbit, or a dog, or rat, or the other usual test animals. Accordingly, there is always the danger that even with the most vigorous testing we may still get side effects in man that are worse than what we are trying to correct. Further, if the parents volunteer and there is a mistake made, the child pays the price.

Suppose you did volunteer for gene manipulation and there was a side effect, could you face your child? Suppose you didn't volunteer and your defective trait showed up in your child, what then? This is one of those "damned if you do, damned if you don't" situations. Suppose science could really perfect this technique so that one could specify even before conception every attribute of a child—size, shape, I.Q., color, etc. How many parents would vote to "dial-a-child"? Probably few would, so let me pose one more question. Parents work hard to give their children the best economic and educational starts in life; why not the best genetic start in life?

Although in most cases we have to wait until the first defective child is born before we know that the parents are carrying hidden recessive genes, it is now possible to perform reasonably accurate tests prior to marriage to see whether prospective parents are carrying a hidden gene for muscular dystrophy, cystic fibrosis, PKU, galactosemia, certain kinds of diabetes, one type of Mongolism, and the RH blood factors. Research is being carried on so that in the very near future parents may be able to have tests for a hundred defective genes prior to conception.

Continuing our questioning, how many would want such information? Suppose it was found that the prospective marriage partners had matching defects. Should they go ahead and get married? Should they have children? Should it be left strictly to the parents to decide whether they will or will not have children? Denmark already has a law decreeing that people with certain kinds of defects cannot get a marriage license until they have been sterilized.

These are some of the problems that science cannot solve. These are the problems to which careful ethical and moral consideration must be given. What must we do to put scientific developments to proper use? Who will make the decisions concerning their use?

While there is still time, informed citizens must insist that our public officials discuss these new issues and evaluate their impact on society. One fact revealed by the nuclear-testing controversy is that after the bomb has gone off it is too late to begin discussion. This new biological knowledge is a very big bomb with a very short fuse; and the fuse has been lit! Every time science develops insulin or a treatment for some defect without curing it, we ensure that some people will now be kept alive that previously would not have had children. As a result, the number of defective genes is increasing with each generation. While the new treatments are fine for the generations already here, what about those still to be conceived? One per cent of births (40 thousand to 50 thousand children) every year in this country are so defective that they don't know that they are human beings. Every year another 1 per cent are born so defective that they cannot compete socially or economically. In addition, another 4 per cent are abnormal in some other ways. This is a total of about 6 per cent, or one out of every 17 births. We must face these facts while there is still time.

Once the discussion starts, the extremists must not be allowed to take over. By extremists I mean those who will say that these discoveries are all good or that they are all bad. They are neither. For two thousand years we have asked, "What is man? Why is he here?" Suddenly we must ask ourselves the further question, "What would we like him to be?" Easy answers should be suspect.

Further, it is important that the youth, who must make these decisions eventually, get the proper background and guidance. Why the young? For two reasons: One is a simple matter of timing. History teaches that it takes Western society about 25 years to become alerted to important social problems, and another 25 years to get the job done. Civil rights is a good example. Population control seems to be following the same timetable. Young people now attending high schools and colleges will be in charge when the developments and decisions discussed here come to fruition.

The main reason, however, that today's youths must bear the burden of making tomorrow's decisions is that their elders are ill-prepared to do so. Most of these fundamental questions are approached by them with prejudices that seriously hamper their answers. Let me illustrate by returning to a previous hypothesis: Would you vote today to abort an anencephalic child in the third month of pregnancy? We don't have the capability of such accurate prediction today, but we can wait until that child is born and then know for sure that he is anencephalic. Would you then vote to put that child to death? Further, suppose that we could tell the parents prior to conception, "If you have intercourse tomorrow, you will conceive an anencephalic child." Would you tell those parents, "Don't have intercourse or else take some means to see that the child is not conceived?"

I say, determinedly, "Don't conceive"; raise my hand slowly and doubtfully for abortion at three months; and at nine months plus one day, I say, "Let the anencephalic child live." However, at nine months plus two days, the end result of all three decisions is the same—the child is not there. Wherein lies the difference?

How will the young people find the ethical framework within which to make their decisions? In the last analysis two people must ultimately decide whether they do or do not have intercourse with or without contraception at a given time. Still, it is society that must develop guidelines for those who have difficult decisions to make in the genetic areas. It is urgent that we responsibly address ourselves to these profound moral questions that are emerging from our new scientific discoveries, and it is important that we do so *now*.

CHAPTER 9

HUMAN EXPERIMENTATION

Louis Lasagna

The ethical dilemmas facing both science and the public at large are dramatically exemplified by the problems arising out of human experimentation. It is the purpose of this essay to illustrate these complex and troublesome questions with specific examples from two areas: the field of immunization and that of drug development.

The national polio-vaccine field trials of a decade ago are now generally looked upon as a milestone of scientific and social progress. Poliomyelitis, for centuries a dreaded maimer and killer, is now almost as extinct as the dodo. Because of the Salk and Sabin vaccines, countless children and adults will be spared death or a lifetime of residual paralytic disability. It is thus especially easy to forget the substantial ethical problems posed by these trials.

The field-trial design which was ultimately used, and which clearly demonstrated the benefits of the vaccine, was not arrived at without argument. At one point, it was proposed that volunteers should constitute the treated group, and nonvolunteers the untreated controls. In view of the powerful theoretical disadvantages of such an invalid control group, it is remarkable that such a proposal should have been seriously considered. Why was there any hesitation about a proper trial? While I cannot pretend to know all the reasons, certain facts can be listed as sources of difficulty.

To begin with, there was no longstanding tradition for largescale, double-blind, informed-consent trials in the field of immunology, although a controlled trial had been used to test diphtheria antitoxin in 1918. Second, the experimental subjects were children, a population whose special status as dependent wards poses the question of who can volunteer on behalf of a minor. Third, the trial did not involve *treatment* for the children in the trial—there *are* adequate social precedents for parents and even courts giving consent on behalf of minors for medical or surgical procedures—but rather the *prevention* of a disease which even at its height was extraordinarily rare. Fourth, the vaccine, while generally assumed to be safe, could not be guaranteed free of danger. (In fact, certain batches appear to have produced paralytic polio, a fact that became the basis for successful legal action against one of the manufacturers.)

This list of difficulties, which does not exhaust the problems associated with the evaluation of the polio vaccines, provides a background for discussing the more recent Willowbrook experiments. For fifteen years, Professor Saul Krugman of New York University and his colleagues have been studying the natural history of viral hepatitis, with a view toward preventing it. Technical developments in recent years have made available tests to detect both antigen and antibody for this disease, and set the stage for the ultimate success of the NYU group.

Krugman had observed that boiling for one minute at $98^{0}C$ destroyed the infectivity but not the antigenicity of his MS-2 strain of hepatitis virus. Proceeding from this fact, the NYU team succeeded in preventing viral hepatitis by both active and passive immunization, an exciting accomplishment which rated a front-page story from *The New York Times* on March 24, 1971. Krugman has, however, been bitterly attacked on both sides of the Atlantic for his experiments. Why?

The experiments in question, plus the earlier research which laid the groundwork for the vaccine, were conducted at the Willowbrook State School in Staten Island, New York. Willowbrook, the largest such institution in the country, houses 5,500 mentally retarded adults and children. Its patients live in close contact with each other, and hepatitis has been chronically epidemic there since 1949.

The experiments involved the deliberate administration of hepatitis virus to mentally retarded children—and therein lies the problem. The paragraphs that follow give two sides of the story, one by Krugman and the other by a fierce opponent of clinical research, M. H. Pappworth, the physician-author of *Human Guinea Pigs*. Both were published in the Letters to the Editor section of the *Lancet*, May 8 and June 5, 1971, respectively:

> Dr. Joan Giles and I have been actively engaged in studies aimed to solve two infectious-disease problems in the Willowbrook State School—measles and viral hepatitis. These studies were investigated in this institution because they represented major health problems for the five thousand or more mentally retarded children who were residents. Uninformed critics have assumed or implied that we came to Willowbrook to "conduct experiments on mentally retarded children."
>
> The results of our Willowbrook studies with the experimental live attenuated measles vacine developed by Enders and his colleagues are well documented in the medical literature. As early as 1960 we demonstrated the protective effect of this vaccine during the course of an epidemic. Prior to licensure of the vaccine in 1963 epidemics occurred at two-year intervals in this institution. During the 1960 epidemic there were more than 600 cases of measles and 60 deaths. In the wake of our ongoing

measles vaccine programme, measles has been eradicated as a disease in the Willowbrook State School. We have not had a single case of measles since 1963. In this regard the children at the Willowbrook State School have been more fortunate than unimmunised children in Oxford, England, other areas in Great Britain, as well as certain groups of children in the United States and other parts of the world.

The background of our hepatitis studies at Willowbrook has been described in detail in various publications. Viral hepatitis is so prevalent that newly admitted susceptible children become infected within 6 to 12 months after entry in the institution. These children are a source of infection for the personnel who care for them and for their families if they visit with them. We were convinced that the solution of the hepatitis problem in this institution was dependent on the acquisition of new knowledge leading to the development of an effective immunising agent. The achievements with smallpox, diphtheria, poliomyelitis, and more recently measles represent dramatic illustrations of this approach.

It is well known that viral hepatitis in children is milder and more benign than the same disease in adults. Experience has revealed that hepatitis in institutionalised, mentally retarded children is also mild, in contrast with measles which is a more severe disease when it occurs in institutional epidemics involving the mentally retarded. Our proposal to expose a small number of newly admitted children to the Willowbrook strains of hepatitis virus was justified in our opinion for the following reasons: (1) they were bound to be exposed to the same strains under the natural conditions existing in the institution; (2) they would be admitted to a special, well-equipped, and well-staffed unit where they would be isolated from exposure to other infectious diseases which were prevalent in the institution—namely, shigellosis, parasitic infections, and respiratory infections—thus, their exposure in the hepatitis unit would be associated with less risk than the type of institutional exposure where multiple infections could occur; (3) they were likely to have a subclinical infection followed by immunity to the particular hepatitis virus; and (4) only children with parents who gave informed consent would be included.

The statement by Dr. Goldby accusing us of conducting experiments exclusively for the acquisition of knowledge with no benefit for the children cannot be supported by the true facts.

Saul Krugman

Sir,—The experiments at Willowbrook raise two important issues: What constitutes valid consent, and do ends justify means? English law definitely forbids experimentation on children, even if both parents consent, unless done specifically in the interests of each individual child. Perhaps in the U.S.A. the law is not so clear-cut. According to Beecher, the parents of the children at Willowbrook were informed that, because of overcrowding, the institution was to be closed; but only a week or two later they were told that there would be vacancies in the "hepatitis unit" for children whose parents allowed them to form part of the hepatitis research study. Such consent, ethically if not legally, is invalid because of its element of coercion, some parents being desperately anxious to institutionalise their mentally defective children. Moreover, obtaining consent after talking to parents in groups, as described by Krugman, is extremely unsatisfactory because even a single enthusiast can sway the diffident who do not wish to appear churlish in front of their fellow citizens.

Do ends justify the means? Krugman maintains that any newly admitted children would inevitably have contracted infective hepatitis, which was rife in the hospital. But this ignores the statement by the head of the State Department of Mental Hygiene that, during the major part of the 15 years these experiments have been conducted, a gamma-globulin inoculation programme had already resulted in over an 80 per cent reduction of that disease in that hospital. Krugman and Pasamanick claim that subsequent therapeutic effects justify these experiments. This attitude is frequently adopted by experimenters and enthusiastic medical writers who wish us to forget completely how results are obtained but instead enjoy any benefits that may accrue. Immunisation was not the purpose of these Willowbrook experiments but merely a by-product that incidentally proved beneficial to the victims. Any experiment is ethical or not at its inception, and does not become so because it achieved some measure of success in extending the frontiers of medicine. I particularly object strongly to the views of Willey, "...risk being assumed by the subjects of the experimentation balanced against the potential benefit to the subjects *and* [Willey's italics] to society in general." I believe that experimental physicians never have the right to select martyrs for society. Every human being has the right to be treated with decency, and that right must always supersede every consideration of what may benefit mankind, what may advance medical science, what may contribute to public welfare. No doctor is ever justified in placing society or science first and his obligation to patients second. Any claim to act for the good of society should be regarded with distaste because it may be merely a highflown expression to cloak outrageous acts.

M.H. Pappworth

Two additional points are of interest. Dr. Henry K. Beecher, who has been critical of Krugman's procedures in the past, also wrote a letter to the *Lancet* which was published in the same issue as Pappworth's blast:

Sir,—As one who has had a longstanding interest in human experimentation, I have been troubled by a statement in the otherwise excellent report of the Medical Research Council (*Responsibility in Investigations on Human Subjects,* for 1962-63 [Cmnd. 2382], pp. 21-25), which says: "In the strict view of the law parents and guardians of minors cannot give consent on their behalf to any procedures which are of no particular benefit to them and which may carry some risk of harm." Three years ago I sought the legal basis of this statement. To make the story short, I was finally referred to Sir Harvey Druitt, who said (Dec. 16, 1968), in regard to the above matter, "The statement of the legal position quoted. . .was based on my advice. I am confident about the correctness of that statement, but I cannot cite any statutes or decided case which is exactly in point." (Sir Harvey has generously given me permission to quote him.) I cannot see that a "strict view of the law" is involved.

On a recent visit to the Medical Research Council's headquarters, I was given a reprint of the 1962 statement as currently in force. While some may consider this a trivial matter, I do not believe that it is. Sir Austin Bradford Hill has had some trenchant comments to make against unreasonable restrictions on experimentation in children (*Br. Med. J.* 1963, i, 1043).

As one who has greatly profited over the years from the attitudes and conclusions of the Medical Research Council I would hope that there might be some modification in their stern view of the present matter.

Henry K. Beecher

And in the same issue of *The New York Times* referred to above, New York State Senator Seymour J. Thaler described Dr. Krugman as a "dedicated" and "decent" researcher who "has done a magnificent thing." Four years earlier Thaler had described the children at

Willowbrook as "human guinea pigs." Thaler had also at one time introduced a bill in Albany barring research on children without a court order—a bill which if in effect nationally would have rendered impossible the polio field trials described above. (It is perhaps fair to point out that Krugman had modified the consent procedures originally employed: they had, however, been approved in their earlier form by local, federal and state agencies, as well as a Washington research committee.)

In the area of drug development, different kinds of problems obtain. There are, to be sure, difficulties that revolve around the issue of research subjects under the legal age of consent. Some would oppose the giving of new drugs to children under any circumstances, forgetting that to do so risks the creation of what Shirkey has called "therapeutic orphans." For even if an exciting drug is thoroughly tested and approved for use in adults, there comes a time when the first child has to receive it. For that child, the drug remains "experimental," since no one can be sure whether children will respond the same way as adults, what dose they will require, and so forth.

Let us consider the ethical problems in drug development by tracing a new drug through its career. The very first decision in regard to drug development comes when the animal data are evaluated. Is the drug worth pursuing for human use? The data to support this decision are of several kinds. First, the compound must look therapeutically attractive; that is, it must do something in the laboratory that suggests medical application in man. The other side of the coin is the drug's potential. Does the efficacy: toxicity dosage ratio look favorable?

These matters involve not only scientific but ethical judgments. For instance, a successful diuretic compound or a tranquilizer can command a large market. Many companies, especially those with a significant corps of detail men and effective sales forces, suspect that if they market their own version of such a drug (even if it is not greatly dissimilar from older versions) they can acquire a fraction of the total market. From the consumer standpoint, this may be not much of a gain at all, but the pharmaceutical executive sees it as a way of assuring income to support research on other, potentially more interesting compounds.

In regard to toxicologic data, there are also ethical considerations. How much preclinical toxicity testing is "enough"? To predict extremely rare toxic effects in man—even if a suitable animal model can be found—requires large numbers of animals. By contrast, predicting common toxic effects requires much less expenditures of energy and money. Should all compounds be worked up in thousands of animals, or is the more traditional, less extensive workup adequate? We are faced (as usual) with a cost-benefit analysis, knowing that a compulsively thorough toxicology program (which still won't predict all the trouble to be seen in the clinic) may preclude drug development because of the costs and time involved.

Once the decision is made to give the drug to man, other ethical problems arise. On whom should the drug first be tested? At present, both scientific and regulatory pressures encourage the accumulation of human pharmacologic data that is not therapeutic in nature, but provides information on the absorption, distribution, excretion, and side effect liability of the drug. These experiments are not likely to benefit those first receiving the new chemical, even if the subject is suffering from the disease for which one hopes the drug will be useful. To employ sick patients for these early trials means exposing them to possible discomfort or morbidity, with almost no immediate therapeutic benefit. To use prisoner volunteers, on the other hand, upsets those who believe that sick patients might at least ultimately benefit from the drug's successful development.

This aspect is further complicated by the philosophy popular in some circles that prisoner volunteers can never ethically be used in experimentation. There are, paradoxically, two separate schools that oppose the use of prisoners for different reasons. One group, the "turn-the-screw-a-little-tighter" school, argues that prisoner volunteers may benefit in terms of parole credits, and that they should not be allowed to shorten their prison term in this way. The other group, the "let's not be beastly to the convicts" school, argues that these men are captive in a very special sense, and are more likely to be abused and coerced into volunteering.

Those few prison research setups I have been able to inspect have convinced me that with appropriate safeguards in regard to protocol and to mechanisms for selecting and screening volunteers, there is less risk of coercion in this situation than in most others. Prisoners are usually delighted to volunteer, afflicted as they are with boredom, or guilt, or a yearning for human (and nonprisoner) companionship. Most such drug-research units have more volunteers than they can possibly use, and there is ample opportunity to communicate the purposes and risks of the experiment, with a chance for the volunteer to withdraw either before or at any time during the experiment.

Once a drug has successfully hurdled the earliest human experimentation (which usually serves primarily to indicate what doses are tolerated by healthy individuals), the drug is ready for therapeutic trial. A new ethical dimension now appears. If a drug is proposed to treat a disease or symptom for which no remedy exists, the ethical problems are minuscule. But this situation hardly ever obtains. Usually one or several drugs for the condition already exist, and while they have defects—no drug is perfect—the likelihood of success with one of the standard remedies is reasonably good. In such a situation, how does one justify exposing a patient to a new medicament? If the complaint is a trivial one, and if failure of this new medicament can be ascertained with considerable speed and an effective remedy promptly applied, it may be argued that the patient will be subjected to very little trouble, and that if he is fully informed and gives consent, there are no serious ethical difficulties involved.

This may or may not be true, but the same arguments certainly do not apply to the management of such a serious illness as pneumococcal pneumonia. Here is a condition for which effective remedies exist, remedies whose toxic cost is not excessive. Can one justify the application of a new unproven antibiotic to a patient with pneumococcal pneumonia? It would seem difficult to do so.

The alternative, however, is also not satisfying. It is simply to reserve application of a new remedy to cases in which standard therapy has failed. Any success achieved in such cases is of course highly encouraging, but by definition failure of a drug to perform well in such patients means little or nothing, since the standard drugs have also failed. The possibility therefore exists that a new drug, which may be as good as or better than the old ones, will be missed, and that society will be deprived of a useful remedy.

Similar problems arise in clinical trials where a medication has to be compared against some standard. Even if the ethical difficulties described above have been satisfactorily dealt with, one is still left with the problem of what to compare the new drug against. Shall it *only* be compared against the best available drug, a design which seems both most ethical and most acceptable to the patient? If such a design is pursued, a superior performance of the drug as contrasted with the old is satisfying, but failure of the drug to be distinguished from the standard drug does not necessarily mean anything. It is not uncommon, in certain types of clinical trials, for experimental populations to be fairly insensitive in discriminating between good drugs and bad. A "no difference" result therefore may mean that the new drug is better than the old drug, or as good, or worse! Scientifically, therefore, the more ethical design is not so satisfactory, and in the long run may even prove less ethical, since the marketing of drugs whose merit has not been clearly delineated serves the public poorly.

The problem of consent remains a thorny one. What is truly informed consent? How much information should be given to a subject? What attempts should be made to ascertain whether he fully understands the risks involved? In an experiment we conducted, it was found that potential subjects varied considerably in their understanding of the risks. Furthermore, the degree of comprehension (as well as the likelihood of volunteering) was inversely related to the amount of information presented to the potential volunteers.

Some experiments are difficult or impossible to run if the investigator is fully candid with his subjects. If, for example, one wants to study the effect of the placebo on patient response, informing the patient that he will receive the placebo may destroy (or at the very least modify) the experiment. It is akin to tapping a jury room to listen to the deliberations of the jurors after informing them that the room is "bugged." Some would say that if an experiment cannot be done without fully informed consent, so much the worse for the experiment. Whether this is an ethical stançe or not depends on the point of view, including the question of "statistical morality," that is, whether benefit to large numbers of individuals justifies infringement on the freedom of a few.

A recently criticized study illustrates some of the difficulties. Clinic patients of Mexican-American descent in a Texas city were involved in a study where some of the women received a standard oral contraceptive, while others received a placebo. The women were told that some of them would have to use a medically accepted vaginal cream or foam contraceptive as a backup, because the investigators were not sure whether everyone would receive an effective treatment. (The study was double-blind.) This warning was given to the patients before enrollment in the study, and the importance of using the backup protection was emphasized each month as the patients were brought back to the clinic and personally handed fresh supplies.

As a result of this study, a number of women became pregnant. (The original paper said 11; a later statement by the principal investigator said that there were "only" seven pregnancies in the study.) The majority of the pregnancies occurred in the placebo group, but one woman who was given an active drug but admitted unreliability in taking the medication also became pregnant. All but one of the remaining women who became pregnant while using vaginal cream or foam (plus placebo) "admitted readily to the examiner unreliability in the use of pills and cream or foam."

The investigator argued that if the women had been compulsively scrupulous in their use of the backup contraceptive, few pregnancies would have resulted. This statement is difficult to accept, since almost everyone agrees that oral contraceptives constitute the technique least likely to fail. It is also known that the problems involved in using mechanical devices of one sort or another predispose to unreliability in performance. Scientifically, the investigators could argue that the study was important to define the frequency with which side effects were in truth attributable to oral contraceptives. The study showed that many of the side effects ordinarily linked with the pills are in fact as likely to occur in subjects receiving placebos. This is important information, and one is left arguing whether the scientific insight thus obtained can justify treating a group of women in such a way as almost to guarantee that some in the control group would become pregnant.

There are special problems relating to the mentally disturbed. Psychiatrically ill patients are perhaps more dependent than most patients on a satisfactory patient-doctor relationship. Is is possible for a physician to involve such a patient candidly in an experiment without destroying this relationship? Can one rely on third-party consent for such individuals? How "crazy" is crazy enough not to be able to give permission?

Some, to be sure, would argue that the patient's own doctor should never be the investigator in any clinical trial, but a great deal of drug research is done by physicians who are the primary doctors of record for the subjects. Whether another doctor (or a research committee) can serve as "ombudsman" in these circumstances is a moot point.

A special point of worry is whether the various techniques that have been invoked to safeguard human rights and to generate interpretable experiments have so altered the therapeutic situation as to render generalization of results impossible. Is there enough of a "Heisenberg effect" produced so that the results are quantitatively (or even qualitatively) different from what will be achieved in actual practice? Regardless of the scientific defensibility of experimental strictures, most patients are not treated under double-blind, controlled conditions, and do not have a great deal of discussion with their doctors about the pros and cons of various therapeutic modalities. (This real-life situation may or may not be desirable, but it is a fact.) There is evidence that doctor attitudes may have great therapeutic impact. An enthusiastic physician can make a drug look "better" than it actually is, and an unenthusiastic doctor can detract from a drug's performance. Can we satisfy ethical requirements and yet not destroy the interpretability and applicability of the experimental results?

This brief analysis, admittedly incomplete, may perhaps have illustrated enough problems to indicate why ethical dilemmas are so prominent in the fields of drug and vaccine development.

CHAPTER 10

MEDICAL ETHICS AND PSYCHOTROPIC DRUGS

ETHICAL RESPONSIBILITIES OF PHYSICIANS IN RELATION TO PROBLEMS OF DRUG ABUSE, AND PUBLIC AND GOVERNMENTAL ATTITUDES TOWARDS THE CONTROL OF THE USE OF PSYCHOTROPIC DRUGS.

Mervyn F. Silverman and Deborah B. Silverman

I. ETHICAL CONSIDERATIONS

The medical profession with the foundation of its own principles of ethics, is uniquely qualified to be the guiding force in the cooperative solving of all these problems and in developing national and international ethics, regarding man's future treatment, and perhaps future control of mankind.[1]

—Dwight Wilbur
Former president, A.M.A.

One of the problems to which Dr. Wilbur might well be referring is that of drug abuse. It is interesting to note his belief that the medical profession's ethical heritage gives it special competence to deal with many of society's problems.

When the first written code of ethical principles for medical practice, the Code of Hammurabi, was conceived four thousand years ago, it merely set fees for services and invoked the principle of *lex talionis* (an eye for an eye). In the fifth century B.C. a brief statement of principles, the Oath of Hippocrates, was written advocating the protection of the patient's rights and prescribing ideals of conduct for the physician. In 1803 British physician and philosopher, Thomas Percival, published his *Code of Medical Ethics,* which became the basis of the ethical principles adopted by the A.M.A. when it was founded in 1847. Actually, the *Code* was concerned not with ethics but with etiquette—social conduct based on custom rather than on moral values. As late as 1955, an attempt was made to separate medical ethics from matters of etiquette; it was finally accepted by the Association's House of Delegates in 1957.

Recently, however, Dr. Chauncey D. Leake stated, "What is ordinarily called 'medical ethics,' which is really a matter of decent etiquette, has scarcely ever been concerned with any genuine ethical theory, although social idealism is usually professed by medical apologists, and frank hedonism practiced by members of ths profession."[2] Obviously, a comparison of the comments by Dr. Wilbur and Dr. Leake illustrates a difference of opinion with regard to the profession's qualifications as a "guiding force." But even though organized medicine has been noticeably unprogressive in times of social crisis, certain values are implicit in the very existence of modern medicine as a profession, and in its assumptions as a science.

Before considering these more specific values, let us put them in the more general context of a value theory. Ethics is a discipline in that it is built on a reasoned conception of reality, and based in fact. We arrive at a perspective of what is, and we infer what ought to be; we fashion our conduct in each situation accordingly. Philosophers ancient and modern have concerned themselves with the values of goodness and beauty, and have found the infusion of values in the structure of reality itself.[3] If this were not the case, value theory would be a matter of superstition or mere personal preference. This basis in fact is a key point, because it holds us to the view that ethics is a practical matter, dealing as it does with implications for our conduct, itself the essence of practicality.

The threefold nature of ethics as (1) our basic assumptions, (2) our criteria for choosing goals, and (3) our guide for action will be applied to the problem of drug abuse. For it is necessary to discuss to what degree our society's drug policy is founded in reality, aiming toward a relevant and achievable goal, and progressing in a manner true to those values we profess to hold. The clear implication is that the end never justifies the means, for they are both responsible to the same set of values.

Given this brief ethical scheme, what values does modern medicine assume in its various aspects of practice, research, education, and administration? Medicine assumes the inherent value of human life—indeed, of individual human lives; it assumes the value of basing practice on fact (that is, on knowledge gained by scientific method); and it assumes the value of responsibility or devotion to others. These assumed values operate unnoticed unless there is a challenge to their potentiality for realization: euthanasia, heart transplantation and abortion are, like drug abuse, highly charged issues with controversial ethical implications. The drug abuse situation clearly involves a great potential for human waste, professional negligence, and legislative inconsistency. What is the physician's ethical responsibility regarding this problem? Having discussed our underlying value assumptions, we will devote the remainder of this chapter to some general consideration of drug abuse and its implications for physicians.

II. THE PROBLEM OF DRUGS

Essentially drugs are everything from aspirin to alcohol, caffeine to cocaine, penicillin to "pot," sedatives to stimulants, laxatives to LSD. Today the statement that a person is "on drugs" conjures up visions of someone high on LSD, mainlining heroin, or popping amphetamine pills. In reality all of America is "on drugs." Last year, for example, more than two billion prescriptions were filled in the United States, justifying the statement by the Commissioner of the Food and Drug Administration that "we are an overdrugged nation."[4]

Psychotropic drugs, substances that have their principal effect on mood, thought processes, or behavior, represented approximately 10 per cent or 225 million of the prescriptions written in 1970. It is claimed that in the 12 months which preceded October 1969, as many as one out of four adults took a psychotropic drug; and one out of two had taken at least one at some time in their lives.[5] These drugs include the major and minor tranquilizers, antidepressants, stimulants, sedatives and hypnotics. All have the potential for producing physical and/or psychic dependence except the major tranquilizers (antipsychotic agents), and the antidepressants. More females than males received prescriptions for psychotropic drugs, with the antidepressants and stimulants heading the list (8 per cent of *all* prescriptions written in the U.S.A. are for amphetamines, which are stimulants).

These statistics fall under the category of "drug use," since they describe those drugs legally prescribed by a physician for his patient. Another aspect of the situation is "drug abuse." Many statistical estimates have been made, varying widely in numbers and degree of substantiation. One is that there are approximately 200 thousand narcotics addicts in the United States, 95 per cent of whom are heroin users; 7 per cent are estimated to be under 21 years of age, and 80 per cent are males.[7] The number of physician-addicts has been placed anywhere from 1 to 15 per cent of the total, indicating that drugs are not exclusively a problem of patients.

Although it is sometimes believed that the drug abuse problem is mainly found among the unemployed, a study showed that 53 per cent of business and industrial firms surveyed had discovered drug abuse among their employees.[8] A nationwide poll of college students indicated that 31.9 per cent had tried marihuana, 8.2 per cent LSD, 13.5 per cent amphetamines, and 11.7 per cent barbiturates.[9] One example of the severity of the problem can be seen in New York City, where 1,002 people died of drug-related causes in 1970, and where drug abuse remains the largest single cause of death for individuals between the ages of 15 and 35.[10] (Another sobering statistic is that six thousand deaths in New York City were related to alcohol; yet the state's alcohol rehabilitation programs represent less than 3 per cent of the budget for addict rehabilitation.)[11]

There is much disagreement regarding the accuracy of these statistics, and having reviewed the literature, we are convinced that there is no definitive knowledge of the extent of illegal drug use and addiction. Some figures, derived from hospitals, indicate instances of drug-related health problems; others record mere violation of the law, with no awareness that "drug-use patterns are fluid and that people and circumstances (including drug availability), not the pharmaceutical properties of the drugs alone, determine priorities for drug experimentation and patterns of use among drug-interested persons."[12]

Numerous attempts have been made to define the factors contributing to drug abuse. An experiment conducted at the University of Michigan demonstrated that monkeys, when offered morphine and an inert solution, choose the narcotic. The same results were obtained using psychotropic drugs, even while the monkeys were suffering significant physiological impairment from drug use. As Dr. Louis Lasagna states, "These experiments make one wonder about the analogy between this situation and the frustration, boredom, and sociological imprisonment suffered by many members of society."[13]

Boredom and frustration are not limited to society's underprivileged; the vast majority of our children are subject to physically and intellectually oppressive environments most of their day, while we turn a deaf ear to the carefully reasoned and almost unanimous calls for school reform by experts in the field. As Joel Fort states, "The more we make going to school a mind-expanding experience for young people, the less likely they are to turn to a chemical. Drug use is a symptom of widespread alienation, which includes great dissatisfaction with schools which are increasingly experienced as boring and irrelevant by millions of our young people."[14]

Again, some consider the draft and the Vietnam war major causes of America's drug problems. The disillusionment of youth with a government that sends its young men abroad to die for ideals that are being practiced neither there nor domestically could in itself be the subject of an entire monograph. This same government is working on a national policy statement, a draft of which warns that marihuana smoking could lead to heroin adiction (actually, it has been estimated that only 2 per cent of those who tried marihuana have gone on to heroin, and only one-half of these have become heroin addicts),[15] birth deformities, brain dislocations, bad school grades, "drinking, smoking, and early or steady dating." The draft also states that marihuana smoking is "a defiant act against the 'Establishment.' It is the drug of choice, though illegal, perhaps because it is illegal, of groups which span the whole spectrum of dissent and protest." The Department of Defense states not only that marihuana use is dangerous, but that "there may be very definite and substantial detrimental effects on both the mental and physical well-being of the individual."[17]

Contradicting the above statements is another government publication which states that "The psychological effects of marihuana are variable. More often the feeling is one of a passive euphoria or 'high'."[18] The National Institute of Mental Health has stated: "Physiological changes accompanying marihuana use at typical levels of American social usage are relatively few. Neurological examinations consistently reveal no major abnormalities during marihuana intoxication."[19]

The disillusionment produced by the government's conflicting and hasty reports is intensified by its irrational actions, an example is the Federal Communications Commission's threat to radio and TV station owners that they might have trouble obtaining license renewals if they played songs whose lyrics tended "to promote or glorify" drugs—not the myriad advertised by the media, but heroin, LSD, marihuana, and so forth.[20]

Public disillusionment also extends to the medical profession. At a news conference in March 1971, the president-elect of the American Medical Associaion, Dr. Wesley Hall, stated that marihuana could cause birth defects or loss of sex drive. In response to the reactions to his statements, he commented that he had made no immediate effort to correct the report because he thought it would be a good idea to discourage the use of marihuana. "We're talking about the morality of our country and the loss of respect for law and order and authority and decency."[21] He later stated that "The A.M.A. knows of no evidence to substantiate the statement that marihuana use leads to birth defects and sexual impotence."[22]

In his treatise "The Morality of Medicine," John G. Archer, M.D., remarked, "Our judgment is never better than our information. To make informed judgments, we must possess the necessary knowledge and the ability to use it. This we call wisdom."[23] Neither the government nor the A.M.A. has shown much evidence of such wisdom. They have failed those who might benefit from public education regarding drugs; it is impossible to take such "educational" material seriously, and very easy to disregard it completely. People determined to "turn on" in any case will certainly not be swayed even to do so with moderation and good judgment if the well-earned credibility gap is not closed.

The overproduction of drugs has also been offered as a possible factor contributing to drug abuse. American drug companies have been producing eight billion amphetamines yearly (or 40 for every man, woman, and child in the U.S.A.). According to F.D.A. reports half of them are illegally dispensed. The House Crime Committee cites this overproduction as a cause of amphetamine abuse.[24] Senator Frank Moss (D-Utah), chairman of the Senate Consumer Subcommittee, feels that over-the-counter-drug advertising has "fertilized the social ground in which drug abuse takes root," promising instant gratification through the swallowing, tasting, touching, hearing, and even the smelling of an extraordinary variety of material goods."[25]

The drug industry spends a larger percentage of its income on advertising than is spent by all other industries, regardless of the type of product or service. These ads for public consumption are convincing and clever; they appeal to our hopes and condition our attitudes. Nicholas Von Hoffman asks, "If these drugs are a necessity, if they are so good for us, why should they have to be advertised so?"[26] In addition, physicians, through journals and medical magazines, are confronted by advertisements for prescription drugs to relieve the relatively minor anxiety situations often encountered in the normal day's activities, such as "not fitting in." (The F.D.A. recently took action against a drug company for the "false and misleading implications" of its advertisements.) General reliance on drugs, as well as the typical medical education, has led to overprescribing. It is estimated that by 1975, three billion prescriptions will be written per year. Recent surveys have shown that a patient generally receives about 10 different drugs per hospital admission and that 5 per cent of all admissions to hospitals in America are the result of some form of drug reaction.[27]

Finally, it has been theorized that a leading reason for drug abuse is the lack of a natural development of social controls surrounding nonmedical drug use. While we have incorporated into daily life the rituals and social amenities regarding other behavior (the cocktail hour limits alcohol use by expressing the notion that drinking is not a solitary activity), we have placed casual drug use outside the bounds of acceptable social behavior. While use itself is not necessarily an illness, any more than is the use of alcohol (or even food), medical help is sometimes necessary when controls regarding the use of any of these substances fail to relate to an individual's life. Whatever people use, some will abuse; such abuse—of drugs, alcohol, food—may stem from personal problems, and can result in damage to health.[28]

But determination on the part of many to "turn on" in one way or another must gradually be recognized as part of life's reality if our society is to be accepting and supportive of its individuals. "When the mores are adequate, laws are unnecessary; when the mores are inadequate, the laws are ineffective."[29]

III. THE LAWS

The laws, with their ramifications, are a central part of the drug problem. In his book *The Addict and the Law,* Alfred R. Lindesmith documents the legislation concerning drugs, and its step-by-step elimination of the doctor's role in controlling the effects of drug misuse and in making drugs available to addicts. By 1922, physician involvement was virtually prohibited and drug addiction had become a criminal offense. Subsequent court decisions were reactive and piecemeal, and created a wholly self-contradictory state of affairs. Even today, "the physician has no way of knowing *before* he attempts to treat, and/or prescribe drugs to an addict, whether his activities will be condemned or condoned. He does not have any criteria or standards to guide him in dealing with drug addicts, since what constitutes bona fide medical practice and good faith depends upon the facts and circumstances of each case. . ."[30] The court decisions, as a body of policy, in effect discourage concerned action; ignoring the physician's professed motives and expertise, the court rules on his knowledge and good will.[31]

Unfortunately, drug laws have often grown out of emotionalism rather than sound scientific research. This is evidenced in the reaction to LSD in 1966: Within a period of four months, the government outlawed the manufacture, distribution and sale of LSD; New York State made it illegal to carry it or give it away; legislation banning it was pending in four other states; the only legal manufacturer stopped experiments on it; and three Senate subcommittees investigated the LSD "problem."[32] We are still ignorant about LSD. It has now been pushed underground, but it will never be legislated out of existence as long as someone is willing to pay the price for it.

It is apparent that the laws pertaining to drugs are basically unenforceable and fail to control drug behavior. As we should already have learned from Prohibition, the effects of unenforceable laws are negative, "through their influence on the social meanings read into various acts or behavior patterns, and through their role in structuring total problem situations."[33]

The addict's "problem structure" is a spiraling pattern of increasing involvement with drugs. Schur flatly states, "The practical effect of American narcotics laws is to define the addict as a criminal offender."[34] Added to his need for drugs is the need to act like a criminal in order to get them. Soon he is committing offenses to acquire money for drugs, and setting up continuing associations with the underworld to obtain the emotional and practical support he now requires. "Here surely is a clear illustration of a basic sociological theme: the nature of an individual, as he himself and we impute it to him, is generated by the nature of his group affiliations."[35]

Meanwhile, a successful operation of illegal traffic serves the drug abuser and the addict, with no consumer controls or price ceilings. It is a complex deviant subculture in which the addict is often cheated, law enforcement is thwarted, the traffic cannot be stopped, and the victim cannot complain. Those who stand to gain the most from the illicit drug traffic take the least risk, at the expense, of course, of the addict.

The effects of unenforceable law are evident not only in the underground; society at large ultimately pays in the form of increased crime, taxpayers' money for law implementation, loss of human resources, and the infusion of corruption into our law enforcement agencies. Such corruption in the enforcement of present drug laws, cited in studies by Shur, Blum, and Lindesmith, involves the assumption of false identity, entrapment, and the selective rewarding of informants with money or drugs. Invasion of privacy, search and seizure, and the "no-knock" policy, all violate the constitutional rights of innocent and guilty alike. Add to this the inevitable bribery, blackmail and brutality. In the middle is the addict, who is doubly vulnerable—to his suppliers and associates, and to the police.

An outgrowth of our irrational policy is what amounts to cruel and unusual punishment, out of all proportion to the offense. Two years ago, 300 thousand people, many in their 20's or younger, were arrested on felony charges for possession or sale of marihuana. Presently there are over 200 thousand serving sentences up to and beyond 20 years. In short, "The laws breed their criminals, turning the young of America into an outlaw class."[36]

Many of these ills demonstrate the lack of application to any ethical standard. To refer to our threefold scheme of ethics, present policy has not (1) taken cognizance of underlying, governing *facts* and *values*, or (2) aimed at the achievement of a reasonable *goal* in keeping with those values. (3) It is especially noteworthy that the *process* of implementing the policy has failed to exemplify the principles expressive of these values.

Yet the President's Task Force Report on Narcotics and Drug Abuse (1967) recommended that this battle between underground and establishment be escalated, with increases in funds and manpower, while ignoring the unenforceability of the laws, the effects of punitive measures, and the rapid multiplication of drug and drug-related problems. This they do even in the face of their own admissions that smuggling can never be completely prevented, that the scarcity of drugs produces more profits for traffickers and greater desperation among addicts, and that efficient punitive control, if at all possible, would involve policies oppressive to everyone.

In effect, policy-makers, their advisers, and large numbers of apathetic and mute professionals have assigned to law-enforcement officials the impossible task of managing an unmanageable problem: that of eradicating personal need and controlling private transactions between consenting persons. The officials done their best to devise methods to carry out the law and cater to public fear. But inadequate laws cannot conceal real social ferment. On the contrary: "Unenforceable criminal law serves as an indicator of inconsistencies in a society's value system; it may reveal conflicts of interest. . .underlying the legal structure and may serve to pinpoint significant loci of change."[37]

IV. UNDERSTANDING DRUG-ABUSE CONCEPTS

Change requires new thinking, and our first step is to divest the language relating to the problem of its ambiguities and prejudices. What is meant by the word "abuse" (compared to "use") and "addict" (as opposed to "user")? What do we mean by labeling a drug "dangerous," and what harm, primary and secondary, do we fear?

The primary concern is with addiction itself. It is hard to imagine what our practical objection to drugs would be if they were not potentially addicting, mind-altering, or in some way destructive of our mental or physical health. But what is addiction? The Task Force Report tells us:

> There is no settled definition of addiction. Sociologists speak of "assimilation into a special life style of drug taking." Doctors speak of "physical dependence," an alteration in the central nervous system that results in painful sickness when the use of the drug is abruptly discontinued; of "psychological or psychic dependence", an emotional desire...and of "tolerance", a physical adjustment to the drug that results in successive doses producing smaller effects, and, therefore, in a tendency to increase doses. Statutes speak of habitual use; of loss of the power of self-control respecting the drug; and of effects detrimental to the individual or potentially harmful to the public morals, safety, health, or welfare.[38]

The notion of addiction does not suggest the degree or type of dependence, nor does it define the field of drugs involved. But addiction is the extreme within the total drug scene. Some drug abuse involves the misuse of legal drugs, and the mere use of illegal ones. Almost everyone, as we have said, has taken a psychotropic drug.

But with regard to drug abuse itself, our concepts are even less helpful. They do not include notions of what drugs, dosages, circumstances, or purposes are appropriate; they do not suggest what results, objective or subjective, justify use. Much socially condoned drug usage is really misuse, in that it is not demanded by a condition, not effective for a particular condition, or not safe enough to warrant the risk. Drug classification, legal and popular, is irrational and inconsistent in ways that speak to almost every one of us: "While the use of marihuana is illegal, the use of alcohol is not, even though alcohol produces physical dependence and is addicting in the same sense that heroin is, while marihuana is not an addicting drug. The reader might well ponder what the effects would be if alcohol were handled as heroin is and if alcoholics were subjected to the treatment accorded opiate addicts."[39] Alcohol, aside from its lack of medicinal utility and its association with dependence, has been associated with organic disorders, and often with violent or irresponsible behavior. Opiates have not yet been associated with any physiologic disorders, and are not in themselves responsible for violence.[40] The possibility of addiction and the felt effects of the drug depend largely on the individual and his situation.

Still, there are greater similarities between alcohol and heroin than between marihuana and heroin, even though the latter two have been seen as equivalent in the eyes of the law. Experts have repeatedly urged a separate classification for marihuana, on the ground that its threat to society and to the individual is probably much less than that of alcohol. There is no scientific basis for assuming that marihuana use leads to heroin use, nor any justification for the severe penalties imposed for it. Fortunately, we are now beginning to see a change in the legal treatment of marihuana use.

The misuse of barbituates, a socially approved drug, involves the possibility of dependence and tolerance, and even death through overdose or use in combination with alcohol. "Unlike the opiates, such as heroin, the serious consequences of misusing barbiturates are mostly related to the drug itself and not to how the person gets it into his system or his general way of living."[41] What seems clear is that we have not classified drugs with any sense of their potential physical harm, their psychic effects, or people's desire or determination to use them.

As with drugs themselves, our characterizations of the drug user (and pusher) are based on myth. Social mobility, not so much in class as in life-style, has blurred the distinctions that link a social problem with one group and not another. "Dope fiends" are college students and ghetto youth, professionals and vagrants. The woman in labor, along with her unborn child, receives potent drugs; hyperactive children are given amphetamines to make them more amenable to classroom control, the housewife is given a prescription for tranquilizers to make her better able to accept and function in the role society has carved out for her. It seems that the vast majority of this type of drug usage is unnecessary from a medical standpoint, and is simply, like much illicit drug use, the attempt to obtain relief. And often the degree of involvement with the law varies according to the socioeconomic and political status of those concerned. But whoever uses drugs illegally faces the possibility of a head-on collision with society, and an interpretation of his activities which can stigmatize him and set up a pattern for his life.

Because the effects of drugs vary according to (1) the person and (2) his circumstances, we should switch our attention to these two factors. In turning to the persons, we touch on what is very likely our most widespread fear regarding the drug problem. For,

> we would propose that people are worried about people, not about drugs except as these are a mirror reflecting distress. What people are said to do because of drugs—to rob and steal and rape, to injure and kill one another on the highways, and to become dependent and psychotic—these are the things that people do and we—all of us—have a good reason to be upset about them. But people do not need drugs to act in these frightening and damaging ways; and the general evidence is that drugs in fact play a very

> small part in the production of our overall rates of trouble. They do play some part of course and insofar as they do they add to the already great social burden.[42]

Drugs are playing an ever more dominant social role, but even as their effects increase "it is more important to focus on the person than the drug. . .more reasonable to find the motivation in the psyche than in the chemicals."[43] A nonhumanitarian solution to this human problem is no solution at all.

In focusing on the *circumstances* of drug use, we find that the differences between an approved and a disapproved environmental situation affect the quality of the activity itself. Relief is sought in the habitual ways—either through socially approved institutions that are accessible, understandable, and familiar, or in other ways that are relevant and comfortable for the individual. Money, education, location, living conditions, and marginality to the dominant culture all are contributing factors in determining what choices are open. In unapproved settings, drug use does not relate to other aspects of life; social control and standardization of behavior is lacking. But "when drug use begins and is learned within approved and controlled settings and continues in those culturally integrated settings, individual variability in response to drugs is low (that is, most people can be expected to act in the ways the institution expects them to act)."[44]

Taken together, the foregoing observations imply that the resolution of the drug problem is tied into the solution of more basic social problems. Toward this end, we need a liaison of law, medicine, and sociology. Secondly, if the difference between use and abuse is the setting, a matter of social approval and control, then we must accept the responsibility for such control by switching the entire complex of drug activities over to approved institutions. In providing drugs, treatment, the opportunity for cure—all in the proper setting—we gain predictability and factual knowledge, we salvage human resources, we undermine the structure of the criminal drug subculture, and we gain an increment of the humanity and ethical commitment that are increasingly missing in our society.

V. GENERAL POSSIBILITIES FOR SOLUTIONS

Are there any indications that the problems of drug abuse and addiction would respond to a different policy? One alternative is the system practiced by Great Britain, in which secondary problems have largely been avoided by making drugs available when needed on a low-cost basis. "The British program with respect to addicts is in reality absurdly simple and almost impossible to misunderstand. The addict simply goes to a doctor, confides in him, and is taken care of by the doctor. The latter is under a professional obligation to attempt to cure the addict, but there is no provision for forced cures."[45] The illicit market is largely undermined; the addict can avoid stigmatization and harassment. While humane and oriented toward the individual, this program benefits all of society in terms of safety and economy. It is not without problems, and even serious failings, according to Dr. Max M. Glatt, British expert on drug abuse. But in the absence of a perfect solution, research into a possible modification of the British program is called for. (In fact, research of this kind is presently going on for a possible pilot program for New York.)[46]

A second indication for policy change is the fact that doctor-addicts in our country are not associated with criminal or subculture activities. Because they can obtain needed drugs without devoting their lives to the effort, they easily avoid criminalization and can carry on useful activities. By contrast, "The gradual immersion of most American addicts in a world of their own is inextricably connected with the general process by which they have been cast out of respectable society."[47]

Both these examples suggest a rationale for medical provision of all drugs. In this situation, doctors would not necessarily be condoning drug misuse, any more than they demonstrate approval of any form of self-abuse by treating its results. Controlled treatment offers the possibility of eventual cure and provides factual knowledge gained from collective experience.

> Until recently the addict had few public spokesmen while the repressive, antiaddict attitude received strong support from public officials. Indeed, some critics argued that these officials had developed a vested interest in existing policies. In a sense, the medical profession also benefitted from such policies, which relieved the profession of the burden of responsibility for dealing with addiction. Inability to effect easy and lasting cures, and the well-known fact that addicts are extremely difficult patients, may have contributed to medical ambivalence toward drug-law reform.[48]

It is true that the law has worked against even the concerned physician, by limiting his professional freedom to treat drug patients. Moreover, the class of drug users has been remote from professionals, and unable to seek care intelligently or to pay for it. Today these circumstances are changing. Doctors work not only in clinical practice, but in policymaking positions, in public health, in education, and in multidisciplinary, socially oriented organizations, full and part-time. This greater diversification of medical human resources makes advancement possible. What we have suggested so far is a return to the realities of the drug situation: to the basic categories of people (drug users), settings (approved and appropriate environments), and now, of treatment (in the sense of "caring for").[49] Treatment is primary, for cure is possible only for a willing, cooperative patient, one who is not frantic about his ability to receive needed drugs, or hostile toward society for preventing him from getting them. "The exclusive emphasis on complete cure of individual cases and on total elimination of addiction has hindered treatment experimentation and other policy reforms. . .Despite pious protestations, it seems clear that. . .repressive policies. . .represent societal decisions as to how the various demanded goods and services are to be allocated."[50] The New York Academy of Medicine, as early as 1955, demonstrated its agreement with this appraisal of the situation, stating "We are not saying to give the addicts more drugs. We are simply advising a different method of distribution. . .Every addict gets his drugs right now. . .why not let him have his minimum requirements under licensed medical supervision, rather than force him to get it by criminal activities, through criminal channels?"[51]

We need to realize that eradication is an unrealistic goal, so that we can settle down to a constructive, long-term solution. Society, like the drug abuser, must stop believing in the magic of any single cure for its problems, and institute a sane complex of effective measures. Any action in the name of moral values is empty principle if it is not based on the facts. "The more constructive sociological task is to try to understand the behavior in its relation to human needs and social values and institutions, and to help decision-makers determine which policy will best maximize social gains and minimize social costs."[52] Ethical activity means making choices to minimize the evils of a situation and magnify the goods.

VI. ETHICAL RESPONSIBILITIES OF PHYSICIANS

"Any effort to modify present programs by developing new social policy must expect to follow the time-honored, practical, American legislative process of (a) generating pressure for change, (b) participating in the debate over those changes, and (c) finally accommodating to a compromise. . ."[53] We need new facts, strong pressure groups from the ranks of concerned professionals, and education of public opinion. Physicians are directly implicated in the initiation of this process, with their already powerful medical lobby, their special interest groups, and their individual expertise. Such a cause relates to medical educators, researchers, and public-health doctors; perhaps a new class of paramedical personnel could be created to meet the needs arising from the new system.

In mapping out a probable plan for reform, Lindesmith notes that "the first point of attack should probably be the regulations of the Treasury Department which threaten the physician with criminal prosecution for prescribing drugs for users."[54] In gaining the legal right to care for addicts and others with drug problems, the doctor would simply be acting in his traditional role of giving support and relieving unnecessary suffering by extending his characteristic handling of drugs. (Doctors often prescribe drugs to treat symptomatic conditions, with or without any demonstrable physiological malfunction.) Such legal reform should, of course, stress the right of doctors to respect the medical code of confidentiality. Sponsoring legal revisions would also serve the cause of public education, since laws often condition public opinion.

Aside from this, the physician must support reform in practice, where it is directly relevant to the real-life situation. We live what we believe, or else we live in apathy. And even apathy pales in the light of hostile actions by a few physicians. One recent example in our own community is that of a Maryland physician whose home and office are near a proposed "halfway house" for a small number of teenagers who have drug problems but are not addicts. His opposition to the planned rehabilitation center is apparent in his statement to the press: "I told my wife if this thing goes through I thought we should get our shotgun loaded."[55] Contrast this to Dr. Harry F. Dowling's conception of a physician's responsibility: "...we must expect more of doctors than men of any other calling. Compared with other professions, their training is the longest; they are more highly selected than most, and their actions affect the health, happiness and life of everyone at one time or another."[56]

Many physicians are sincerely concerned about how best to help individual addicts while serving the public interest. A good illustration of this dilemma is methadone treatment. A great deal of controversy is now raging about whether addicts might sell their methadone allotment and perhaps spread addiction. (It is estimated that in Britain, where private physicians can prescribe the drug, at least 600 non-heroin addicts have become addicted to methadone.) The obvious solution, and one used by most clinics in this country, is to dispense one dose at a time, to be taken in the clinic or office. This does little for the patient's self-image and can hamper his ability to hold a job. Unfortunately, local medical societies and federal and local narcotic authorities have campaigned to eliminate the private physician as a source of methadone. This could stop treatment for those without a clinic in their community, and allow for the invasion of the patient's privacy.

But legitimate questions are asked about methadone by those who fear its potential long-range effects and by those who feel that methadone treatment will transform a social problem into an individual dilemma that will be easier for society to ignore. Some doctors, however, consider it the drug of choice for heroin addiction at present. These concerns demand careful consideration: We must seek factual answers while doing the best we can for addicts.

A doctor's ethical responsibility also demands honesty in researching and reporting the effects of drugs, and honesty with patients. Since it often means taking extra time to give a full and factual explanation and to examine the deeper causes of problems, this is a difficult requirement. Respect for the patient as a complex and intelligent person means that the physician must be able to admit it when he does not know. The doctors has often maintained an air of secrecy and magic, sometimes chiding his patient for venturing a diagnosis or asking too probing a question. As such, he has fallen far short of his potential as an educator in preventative medicine either on a social or on a personal basis. He has sometimes failed to inspire confidence, understanding, and honesty in his patient.

Drug companies, who advertise to doctors, understand this mysticism fostered by the medicine men, and cater to this tendency by offering magic cures (drugs) for complicated psychophysical problems. One drug, a simple combination of aspirin and antacid, is promoted as advantageous in that it is advertised only to the physician, and not to his patient. This advertising would not last a day if doctors did not allow it. The doctor must be careful not to condone in practice what he condemns in theory. Overprescribing—promiscuous use of drugs to solve problems—is drug abuse. Again we insist that consistency is an ethical matter—a matter of responsibility that often involves passing up the easy solutions.

We are not proposing any new ethical principles, but hold to the classic human and professional values. There are no ideals that are not rooted in actual conditions or facts, and we must be responsible to those; that is, we must be consistent, scientific, and honest. We all have a responsibility to our patients and to society at large, although we are involved in different aspects of the problem. But ethically, the appeal is to a very basic level of conscience, to the feeling for the other that is the very basis of medicine. It is expressed in the golden rule, and also expressed in the A.M.A.'s *Principles of Medical Ethics:*

The honored ideals of the medical profession imply that the responsibilities of the physician extend not only to the individual, but also to the society where these responsibilities deserve his interest and participation in activities which have the purpose of improving both the health and well-being of the individual and the community.[57]

References

1. D.L. Wilbur, "The Heritage of Hippocrates," *Journal of the American Medical Association*, 208 (July 28, 1969). p. 841.
2. C.D. Leake, "Theories of Ethics of Medical Practice." *Journal of the American Medical Association*, 208 (May 5, 1969). pp. 842-847.
3. A.N. Whitehead discusses the infusion of values in fact in *Adventures of Ideas* (New York: New American Library, 1962) pp. 150 ff, 163, 211, 251 ff, 279 ff.
4. "How Safe is Your Food?" *U.S. News and World Report* (April 19, 1971), p. 53.
5. M.B. Balter and J. Levine, "The Nature and Extent of Psychotropic Drug Usage in the United States," *Psychopharmacology Bulletin*, Vol. 5, No. 4 (October 1969), pp. 3-13.
6. *Parade Magazine*, February 7, 1971, p. 20.
7. L.G. Richards and E.E. Carroll, "Illicit Drug Use and Addiction in the United States," *Public Health Reports*, Vol. 85, No. 12 (December 1970), pp. 1035-1039.
8. *American Medical News*, April 5, 1971, p. 14.
9. *Newsweek*, December 29, 1969, pp. 42-45.
10. *New York Times*, March 11, 1971.
11. *New York Times*, March 19, 1971.
12. R.H. Blum, *Mind-Altering Drugs and Dangerous Behavior:* Narcotics, Task Force Report: Narcotics and Drug Abuse (Washington, D.C.: Government Printing Office, 1967), p. 53.
13. L. Lasagna, *Life, Death and the Doctor*, (New York: Alfred A. Knopf, 1968), p. 296.
14. J. Fort, *Drugs: For and Against* (New York: Hart Publishing Co., Inc. 1970), p. 150.
15. Even assuming the figures are higher, no cause and effect relationship is indicated by studies to date.
16. J. Anderson, "Policy Draft Links Pot to Early Dating," *Washington* Post (December 16, 1970).
17. Department of Defense, *Directive #1300.11* (October 23, 1970).
18. A Federal Source Book: *Answers to the Most Frequently Asked Questions About Drug Abuse* (Washington, D.C.: Government Printing Office, 1970).

19. *Marihuana & Health: A Report to the Congress from the Secretary, Department of Health, Education, & Welfare,* (Washington, D.C.: Government Printing Office, January 31, 1971).
20. N. von Hoffman, "Complex Persecution," *Washington Post* March 29, 1971).
21. *Evening Star,* April 25, 1971.
22. *American Medical News,* April 12, 1971, p. 14.
23. J.G. Archer, *The Morality of Medicine,* Medical Ethics and Discipline Manual, American Medical Association (1965).
24. *Parade Magazine, loc. cit.*
25. F. Moss, Senator (D. Utah), introducing S1753—Bill to Establish a National Institute of Advertising, Marketing, and Society. Given to the Senate May 3, 1971.
26. N. von Hoffman, "Low Grade Ailments, Patent Medicine—and *Advertising," Washington Post,* April 14, 1971.
27. "How Safe is Your Food," *loc. cit.*
28. This and other insights were called to our attention by Dr. Michael Brown, Associate Professor of Sociology, Queens College, New York.
29. E. Sutherland & D. Cressy, *Principles of Criminology,* 6th edition (Philadelphia: J.B. Lippencott Co., 1960), p. 11; quoted in E. Schur, *Crimes Without Victims: Deviant Behavior and Public Policy* (Englewood Cliffs, N.J.: Prentice-Hall, Inc. 1965) p. 7.
30. American Bar Association and American Medical Association. *Drug Addiction: Crime or Disease?* Interim and Final Reports of the Joint Committee of the American Bar Association and the American Medical Association on Narcotic Drugs (Bloomington: Indiana University Press, 1961), p. 78; quoted in E. Schur, *op. cit.* p. 133.
31. For a more detailed discussion of the paradoxical situation of the legal policy that in one breath allows and in another forbids doctors to relieve conditions consequent to addiction, see A.R. Lindesmith, *The Addict and the Law* (New York: Indiana University Press, 1965), p. 13.
32. J. Cashman, *The LSD Story* (Greenwich, Conn: Fawcett Publications, Inc., 1966) pp. 114-118.
33. Schur, *op. cit.*, p. 7.
34. *Ibid,* p. 130.
35. E. Goffman, *Stigma: Notes on the Management of Spoiled Identities* (Englewood Cliffs, N.J.: Prentice-Hall Inc., 1963) p. 113.
36. M. Rossman, *Drugs: For and Against* (New York: Hart Publishing Co., Inc., 1970), p. 221.
37. Schur, *loc. cit.* p. 7.
38. *Task Force Report: Narcotics and Drug Abuse* (Washington, D.C.: Government Printing Office, 1967), p. 1.
39. Lindesmith, *op. cit.* pp. xx-x.
40. *Ibid.*, p. xi.

41. *Newark Sunday News*, April 18, 1971.
42. R.H. Blum, *Mind-Altering Drugs and Dangerous Behavior: Dangerous Drugs*, Task Force Report: Narcotics and Drug Abuse (Washington, D.C.: Government Printing Office, 1967), p. 32.
43. Lasagna, *loc. cit.*
44. Blum, *Mind-Altering Drugs and Dangerous Behavior: Narcotics*, p. 42.
45. Lindesmith, *op. cit.*, p. 168.
46. *New York Times*, January 24, 1971.
47. Schur, *op. cit.*, p. 145.
48. *Ibid*, p. 162.
49. Blum, *Mind-Altering Drugs and Dangerous Behavior: Narcotics*, p. 57.
50. Schur, *op. cit.*, p. 176.
51. *Ibid*, p. 151.
52. *Ibid*, p. 178.
53. R.H. Blum, *Drugs, Dangerous Behavior and Social Policy*, Task Force Report: Narcotics and Drug Abuse (Washington, D.C.: Government Printing Office, 1967), p. 69.
54. Lindesmith, *op. cit.*
55. *Washington Post*, April 22, 1971.
56. H.F. Dowling, "The Prescribed Environment," *Saturday Review* (April 3, 1971), p. 60.
57. American Medical Association, *Principles of Medical Ethics*, Medical Ethics and Discipline Manual (Chicago: American Medical Association, 1965), p. vii.

CHAPTER 11

PRISON DOCTORS

ETHICAL PROBLEMS FOR PHYSICIANS IN RELATION TO CRIMINAL JUSTICE

Tom Murton

> I swear by Apollo the Physician and Aesculapius . . . that according to my ability and judgment I will keep this oath and this stipulation.
>
> I will follow that system of regimen which, according to my ability and judgment, I consider for the benefit of my patients and abstain from whatever is deleterious and mischievous. I will give no deadly medicine to anyone . . .
>
> Into whatever houses I enter, I will go . . . for the benefit of the sick and will abstain from every voluntary act of mischief and corruption.

Some 2,400 years ago the Greek physician Hippocrates, called the father of medicine, developed a philosophy of doctor-patient relationships which was later enunciated as the Hippocratic Oath; the oath has been adopted as a creed by the medical profession. There are some indications, especially in the state of Arkansas, that prisoners have been excluded from its provisions.

> LL-1 said that in June, 1963, he got into a fight with a longline rider and was hit on the foot with a hoe. He had been hospitalized for three days when Mr. Bruton [superintendent] came to see him and asked what happened. Mr. Bruton then had him put on a table in

> the prison hospital, belted down with one strap across his chest and one across his legs. The inmate doctor wired him up on the "Tucker Telephone" with one wire to his penis and and another to his big toe. The telephone was cranked five or six times.
>
> Informant FL-17 stated this instrument was designed by Dr. Rollins [former prison doctor] and consisted of an electrical generator taken from a ring-type telephone, placed in sequence with two dry cell batteries, and attached to an undressed inmate strapped to the treatment table at the Tucker hospital, by means of one electrode to a big toe and the second electrode to the penis, at which time, a crank was turned sending an electrical charge into the body of the inmate. [He] stated that several charges were introduced into the inmates of a duration designed to stop just short of the inmate "passing out."
>
> FL-14 confirmed the information regarding the "Tucker Telephone" and furnished this investigator with the name of an inmate who was "rung up" by Mr. Bruton so severely that the Inmate Doctor [Doc Morgan] had to drag Mr. Bruton from the crank of the generator.[1]

Although some prison sources attribute creation of the satanic "Tucker Telephone" to former superintendent Jim Bruton of the Tucker State Prison Farm, it is generally agreed that "credit" for this invention must be given to Dr. A. E. Rollins, the prison physician. Mr. Bruton's claim to fame arose from his perfecting the use of this torture device.

While the deficiencies of the Arkansas Penitentiary System are both legion and well-documented, a brief summary of them is necessary to establish the context of the current discussion. The above extracts from the official state police report give little more than clues to the depths of depravity existing in the Arkansas prisons.

Inmates in these prisons were worked literally from dawn to dark, six or seven days a week, in all kinds of weather, at menial, hard, slave-labor chores. They were housed in 100-man barracks and subject to theft of property, abuse, assaults, and gang rape. Because in Arkansas there is no minimum age for commitment to prison, many 14-year-old boys were housed with older offenders and were therefore subject to almost all conceivable acts of sexual depravity. No underwear, boots, jackets, or gloves were ever issued; food consisted of watery rice or weevils and beans; meat in the form of hog-head stew was received only annually; milk was never provided. At the time of the police investigation in 1966, the inmates were observed to be at least 40 pounds underweight. In order to survive, some stole food, others bought it, and some set traps in the fields to catch anything edible.

When goods and services are not provided by the established order, an informal order emerges to fill the void. In the Arkansas prison system, there were only 29 paid staff authorized to administer three institutions with a total of some 1,500 inmates dispersed across 21 thousand acres of sprawling prison farmland. The lack of sufficient supervisory staff resulted in inmates operating the institutions. They determined all work assignments, granted special favors, merchandised prison commodities, and provided all the guard force. Officials explain to curious visitors that one way to distinguish inmates from employees is to recognize that any person carrying a gun is an *inmate*; employees traditionally are unarmed.

This structure of extensive exploitation relied on fear rather than respect to maintain any semblance of control. Since a system of fear must be enforced by more than the mere threat of violence, it is understandable that a system of brutality evolved. Thus, while Arkansas statutes provided for lashing an inmate 10 times per day with "the hide," a five-foot strap capable of maiming, that official method of discipline was augmented by such illegal, but traditional, techniques as inserting needles under the fingernails, crushing knuckles and testicles with pliers, hitting the inmate with a club, blackjack, or "anything you can lay your hands on," kicking him in the groin, mouth, or testicles—and, of course, by use of the infamous

"Tucker Telephone." A logical extension of such a system of brutality is to threaten people with death. For this threat to be meaningful, it must, from time to time, be implemented.

In January, 1967, Governor Winthrop Rockefeller entered office with a mandate to reform the prison system. He was forced shortly thereafter to remove the superintendent of Tucker State Prison Farm to prevent a "slave revolt" by inmates who were rebelling against prison brutality. I was appointed superintendent of Tucker in February of that year and promoted to head all institutions in January, 1968. I was fired 67 days later for discovering, excavating, and revealing the remains of three inmates allegedly murdered by prison officials at Cummins State Prison Farm.

The preceding cursory account of the Arkansas prison system necessarily, because of its length, raises more questions than it answers. Of the many questions that must be answered, the one that will now be dealt with is among the most important, namely. What has been the role of medical authorities in relation to conditions in the prisons?

As has been indicated, the major torture device used in the Tucker prison was devised by Dr. A. E. Rollins at the time he was prison physician. Presumably, he had been charged with attending to the medical needs of the inmates. During his tenure, one death certificate indicates that an inmate died of malaria; witnesses say the man was trampled to death by a guard on horseback. Another inmate's death was attributed to pneumonia; evidence indicates he died as a result of a beating.

Research of prison records by *New York Times* reporter Walter Rugaber has revealed some interesting facts about prison deaths.[2] In the past 30 years, over 50 men have died of "heart ailments." Forty deaths were listed as resulting from "organic heart disease." Another 29 were simply attributed to "unknown causes."

Similarly, Arkansas Corrections Board Chairman John Haley's research indicates that during several one-week periods, from eight to 10 inmates, all in their 20's and 30's, died of "congestive heart failure." A large number of inmates allegedly have died from "sunstroke," "heat prostration," and "malaria." One inmate died of malaria four days after he wrote to his mother advising her that he was in good health.

Such medical records almost in themselves challenge one's acceptance of their credibility. Moreover, as already illustrated, inmate interviews and other accounts are in sharp contrast to the official version. There is a substantial body of evidence indicating that inmates designated for "elimination" were often committed to the hospital, where the prison physician would allegedly "put them to sleep" by a variety of methods. The death certificates were then falsified to indicate acceptable "natural causes," and the victims would be casually hauled by wagon to the fields, where they were dumped, like so much garbage, into a hole.

There are three institutions that constitute the Arkansas prison system: Tucker State Prison Farm, Cummins State Prison Farm, and the Women's Reformatory. Only one physician serves all three of these prisons, but each has its own infirmary and "medical staff."

The Cummins hospital was always the locus of power for exploiting the inmates. From here, the drug operations were controlled. Medical passes, bed space, and treatment were sold to prisoners who were sick. Here much of the torture, including that which led to death, was carried out. Generally, homosexuals retained control of the hospital and forced those in need of medical help, and who had no funds to pay, to submit to homosexual activities in return for medication. The hospital also provided the only legal escape from hard duty in the fields. For a price, processing of new inmates could be delayed or the files marked "light duty."

The Women's Reformatory is located within the confines of Cummins; it usually houses about 40 female inmates. Our investigation of this institution revealed intolerable conditions. These might be exemplified by the following instances of its "medical-treatment program":

A pregnant inmate had been placed in solitary confinement, an unheated, concrete cell detached from the main building, with no bed, no water, and only a tin can for toilet facilities. She went into labor unattended.

Another inmate complained of being extremely ill, but the prison physician diagnosed her case as "malingering" and prescribed "more work" as a cure. She died in bed that night.

Inmate Ann Shappy gave birth to a baby at the University of Arkansas Medical Center at Little Rock on January 6, 1968. After two or three days, she was transferred to the State Hospital at Little Rock and the baby was left a while longer in the obstetrics facilities at the Medical Center. Mrs. Shappy was returned to the Reformatory on January 23 and reported that at no time during the two and one-half weeks had she been allowed to see her baby. A call to both facilities confirmed that hospital officials had denied permission for her to see her own baby, because, they said, "She is a convict and the Welfare Department is going to place the child for adoption anyway."

We found that the established custom for sick call at the Women's Reformatory was to have the female inmates brought to Cummins hospital, where a male "convict doctor" or attendant would "examine" them—without supervision. Those inmates requiring more intensive "treatment" were transferred to the State Hospital at Little Rock. We noted that many female inmates refused transfer to the Little Rock facility, choosing instead to suffer the consequences. This common but perplexing attitude was readily understood once we discovered that the existing practice was to transport male and female patients together in the back of a closed van. The distance to Little Rock was 85 miles; it was not uncommon for a female patient being transferred to the State Hospital for surgery to be raped en route. All of these procedures were established and implemented with the tacit consent of the prison physician.

Tucker State Prison Farm is much smaller than Cummins and has only a limited infirmary. For obvious reasons, Tucker inmates were reluctant to transfer to the Cummins hospital and chose instead to gamble on the competence of the Tucker "convict doctor."

Most medical services were provided by this inmate, who had had no medical training. He treated minor ills, cuts, and physical disorders by his intuition and experience. He also applied the "Tucker Telephone" when directed to by the superintendent. For a fee, his services were available to all inmates. He also sold medical passes, ran an illegal drug operation, and engaged in other forms of exploitation.

At the time of my appointment in February, 1967, the Tucker infirmary had algae growing on the floor and the electrical wiring had been condemned. Water was piped through the building in gas pipes, and the gas was piped through water lines. Meals for the patients were prepared in the infirmary kitchen under conditions that would not be acceptable on a battlefield.

The only shower was a pipe hanging from the ceiling in the corner of one large cell. Fire-fighting equipment consisted of a box upon which was written the admonition "In case of fire, RUN!"

The Tucker infirmary had been built near a bayou in 1922 (making it the oldest structure in use on the farm) and was surrounded by a levee erected to protect the building from high waters. The protection was not always successful, and after heavy rains, the water inside the infirmary was sometimes a foot and a half deep; fecal material floated around the ward and surgical room. When this occurred, the patients were encouraged to remain in their beds and meals were served by a convict doctor wearing hip boots.

Although this facility could not have met any acceptable medical standards, the State Department of Health had licensed it annually, without the benefit of an on-site inspection, since the building had been converted from a death house to an infirmary in 1948. A requested investigation by health officers resulted in revocation of the license and condemnation of the structure *prior* to inspection of the interior of the building.

The prison physician had authorized the continued use of this inadequate infirmary for 19 years, while attached to a new prison building was a medical facility consisting of space for a ward, an area for offices, and an examination room complete with surgical table, operating lights, and other related equipment. This, however, had been constructed for the sole purpose of examining the corpses of those men exterminated in the adjacent execution chamber. The incongruity of providing modern medical facilities for the dead, when the living were not only subject to unsanitary conditions and exploitation, but to torture on the "Tucker Telephone," somehow eluded the prison physician.

At the time of my appointment the prison physician was Dr. Gwyn Atnip, who followed the usual custom of visiting Cummins hospital half a day, five days a week, and Tucker once a month. His Cummins responsibilities included some 1,300 inmates as well as treatment of the staff and their dependents. His visits to Tucker were to the infirmary only. I could not determine how long it had been since a prison physician had visited Death Row, but its oldest resident declared that he had never seen a doctor and he had been confined there for eight years.

Forty-nine-year-old Luther Bailey had also been on Death Row. He had been convicted of rape; the appellate court had set May 25, 1967, as the date for a new hearing in order to determine whether his purported "confession" had indeed been voluntary. Luther Bailey never got to his hearing. He had complained to Jackie Wood, the convict doctor, of severe abdominal pains for at least three weeks during the latter part of January. The prison physician refused to enter Death Row, and because of security precautions, Bailey was not taken to the infirmary. His condition worsened, but Wood was finally able to convince the prison superintendent that Bailey required emergency treatment. He was taken to the State Hospital in early February and died there, shortly after arrival.

The governor, as required by Arkansas statutes whenever the death of a prison inmate occurs, immediately requested an autopsy. But Dr. George W. Jackson, hospital superintendent, refused to perform the autopsy, because, he argued, the inmate had died in the hospital and not in the prison. Bailey's mother was persuaded by her son's attorney, whom I had contacted, to request an autopsy. Although hospital officials consistently refused to release the autopsy report to the governor, the press reported, on the basis of information from other sources, that Bailey had suffered a ruptured appendix that caused peritonitis and then death. Luther Bailey would not have died had he been given prompt medical attention. He had eluded the electric chair for 10 years, three months, and nine days.

On another occasion, in the spring of 1967, Wood advised the Tucker superintendent that inmate Lewenberger was suffering from appendicitis. He was examined by Dr. Atnip, who diagnosed the problem as pleurisy. The inmate failed to respond to the prescribed treatment; he subsequently collapsed and was taken to the state hospital, where surgery indicated that he had appendicitis.

Dr. Atnip was discharged as prison physician in April, 1967. For providing direct medical services to some 1,500 inmates in the three Arkansas institutions, and for indirect services in supervising related areas, he had received an annual salary of only eight thousand dollars, but the quality of his medical services indicates he was probably not underpaid. In addition, he had a full-time private practice in Pine Bluff and also received 20 thousand dollars a year from Cutter Laboratories for providing nominal supervision of Austin Stough's "blood-sucking" program.

A private blood concession operated at Cummins Prison Farm between September, 1963, and August, 1967; it was run by Dr. Austin R. Stough of Montgomery, Alabama, who was referred to as "the Vampire" by inmates. The plasmapheresis program was explained by Dr. Stough as:

> . . . a process by which blood is drawn from donors, and plasma is extracted and packed cells returned to the donors without loss of cell count. The plasma removed is replaced by saline.
>
> The plasma operation at Cummins provides *one of the few rehabilitation services* at the institutions.[3]

Dr. Stough provided a building, equipment, and staff, and the inmates provided blood. Each donor was paid five dollars a pint. The pint was then sold to Cutter Laboratories for 15 dollars. Of the five dollars paid to the inmate, one dollar was "contributed" to the Inmates' Welfare Fund and another to the Officers' Welfare Fund. No ledger was kept of the latter, but the former account accumulated 73 thousand dollars in "blood money." While these funds were not utilized for the benefit of the inmates, except for token "gate money" upon release, prison officials used the money to purchase cars, tractors, combines, and other commodities.

In 1966 and 1967, an average weekly bleeding amounted to 800 pints. John Haley, prison board member, estimated in April, 1967, that Dr. Stough had profits of at least 300 dollars per day. In 1966, according to state records, his income within Arkansas was 150 thousand dollars. In 1967, according to Alabama records, his income within that state was 500 thousand dollars.

Dr. Stough began his plasmapheresis program in March, 1961, at the State Prison at McAlester, Oklahoma, where he operated for two years. His contract was then voided and the state assumed operation of the program. He began a similar operation at Kilby Prison near Montgomery, Alabama, in December, 1962, and expanded it to institutions at Draper and Altmore in 1963.

Not usually reported by Dr. Stough was the high incidence of infectious hepatitis incidental to his blood programs. Recorded deaths from these and related programs were: one in Oklahoma, one in Arkansas, and four in Alabama.

In addition to the blood programs, Dr. Stough has used prison inmates to conduct an estimated 25 to 50 per cent of all initial drug tests in the United States. The Food and Drug Administration reports that since 1963 he has undertaken 130 investigative studies for 37 drug firms. In May, 1969, after questionable methods of procedure were exposed, the Alabama Board of Corrections ordered these drug studies stopped.[4]

While Austin Stough made his money, all of the conditions discussed above persisted. In addition, the prisons never provided any corrective measures for those inmates with defective vision and Dr. W. E. Hutchison, the prison dentist, never filled teeth—because he was paid by the extraction. He visited Cummins weekly to supervise inmates who made dentures; these were sold to those who needed them for 15 dollars per set. He also visited Tucker, once a month. Dental problems were resolved in the interim by a convict doctor, who would sell aspirin or more potent pain killers to those awaiting the dentist's visit. In extreme cases, an inmate would, in desperation, pay the convict doctor to extract a tooth with a pair of pliers. In such cases, horse anesthetic obtained from a veterinarian was injected prior to the operation, if the inmate could afford it.

In the spring of 1967, a representative of the governor's office posed as an inmate in order to investigate dental techniques. Most of the inmates' complaints were verified at that time. The investigator observed that the dentist dispensed with the formality of washing his hands as he moved from one mouth to another. Dr. W. E. Hutchison, like Dr. Atnip, was dismissed.

Finally, the only alternative to Cummins and Tucker "medical facilities" was the Arkansas State Hospital at Little Rock. Superintendent Dr. George W. Jackson and Dr. Elizabeth Fletcher consistently refused to accept patients from the prisons, even though the hospital had a ward with security facilities that were much stronger than those at either prison farm. In June, 1967, the admissions doctor of the State Hospital refused to accept five inmate patients who had been transferred there by the new prison physician, Dr. Willie Harris. Two of the men had injected lighter fluid intravenously and, according to Dr. Harris, one of them was in danger of losing his life. The reason for denying admission was that the prison officials had not paid for bed space in the past, and medical services to the prison were being discontinued until the delinquent account was paid.

Dr. Edward Barron Jr. was appointed Arkansas prison physician in September, 1967. His subsequent investigations of the Cummins prison revealed that orders for medical supplies had averaged eight thousand dollars a month. He found that drugs were issued by inmates and that the "hospital was the wholesale dispensary for the drugs and narcotics" sold at the prison.[5] He promptly reported his findings to the prison board, stopped the drug ring, and for his efforts was investigated by the Lincoln County Grand Jury, which decreed that it was improper for him to expose medical conditions at the prison.

After the initial flurry of activity, however, improvements in the medical program at the prison appeared to stagnate. Although the salary for his position had been increased to 20 thousand dollars per year, Dr. Barron maintained his private practice and spent only eight hours a week at Cummins. The inmate doctor therefore continued to screen for sick call, forged Barron's signature, admitted and discharged patients, and carried the keys to the drug locker.

Dr. Barron never conducted sick call at Tucker. Tucker patients therefore continued to be transferred to Cummins for examination and treatment. Despite reams of papers constituting a "medical file," conditions provided at best only a facade of professionalism. Frequent discrepancies between medical examination forms and observable phenomena tended to lessen faith and confidence in the quality of medical services. Two inmates transferred to Tucker, for example, were received with files indicating "normal vision." Both complained of poor vision and used this as an excuse for not picking all the weeds from the cotton rows on which they had been working. A staff medical technician examined them and verified that not only did each man have poor vision in one eye, but in each case the other eye was glass!

While a medical doctor generally does not hesitate to acclaim his own expertise, most doctors do not claim infallibility. Most will admit that the human error in diagnosis and treatment will probably never be completely eradicated from medical services.

There are, of course, the small minority of medical practitioners who are no doubt guilty of malfeasance, misfeasance, or malpractice, of gross negligence, incompetence, and other transgressions. The courts and self-policing arms of professional associations, however, tend to weed out many of those who persist in these activities.

Unfortunately, it does seem that more emphasis is placed on formality and bureaucracy than on humanitarian considerations. And the argument that the medical services cannot be continued if monetary compensation is not received is a valid one, although it deals with the means of modern medicine and not with the presumed goal, which is to cure the ill.

The foregoing assessments might be applied in a discussion of the conduct of Arkansas prison physicians. There is ample evidence that one prison physician made simple errors in judgment, another received compensation for questionable medical practices, and hospital officials appeared to be more interested in payment for services than in providing services. These activities are not uncommon and can be defended quite well by knowledgeable spokesmen who can recite philosophical and pragmatic reasons for them. But in the Arkansas experience, is there not a problem of a different dimension?

Arkansas prison physicians have tolerated medieval torture and murder in the prison hospitals. Other medical authorities have aided and abetted the intolerable conditions either by actual involvement or by the conspiracy of silence. There is no record of any voice of protest from medical sources during the past century of prison depravity in Arkansas. It may be understandable, although unjustifiable, that medical practitioners want to ignore deficiencies in their own profession. Still, they could have revealed other brutal prison conditions, while avoiding professional jeopardy. Instead, perhaps through indifference, corruption, or a wish to remain uninvolved, they chose to ignore the situation and merrily attended to the more important tasks of life.

But what of the practitioner who uses his skills and office not to relieve pain, but to inflict pain; to impose anguish rather than assuage it; to kill rather than cure? While the prime responsibility for medical defects in Arkansas obviously lies with the prison authorities, the present article has broader implications than a simple indictment of yet another defect in the notorious Arkansas Penitentiary System.

One might also question the American Medical Association's lack of concern for the treatment of Arkansas prisoners. Does it, too, as some critics contend, devote its energies to protecting rather than correcting incompetence within its ranks? Again, setting aside the obvious need for correcting the practices of the prison physicians in Arkansas, could not a voice have been raised concerning the general treatment of prisoners?

What is the reason for this? Traditionally, the jail or prison physician has had free rein in medical matters. Prison officials do not make it a practice to question his decisions. How then, if the medical officer is committed to lifelong humanitarian service, can he suppress his own goals and ignore the brutality that goes on in most institutions?

As has been suggested, the answer seems to be that there are overriding factors affecting the physician's conduct in these circumstances; for instance, professional survival, advancement, accumulation of wealth, and so on, may pre-empt his oath. But that is not sufficient: It is incongruous that a physician could simultaneously see himself as a part from the system, yet mysteriously demonstrate allegiance to it. For a doctor who treats the wounds of victims of the prison system without speaking against the brutality that caused them becomes an accomplice to the crime. His action, or lack of action, communicates a curious point of view. Thus, given the fact that dismissals of prison physicians for exposing brutality are almost as rare as dinosaurs, one might conclude that there *is* no great internal conflict and that, therefore, for all intents and purposes, the prison physician views the *prison system itself as his client and the inmate-patients as incidental to the relationship.*

Accordingly, could not one argue that the system pays the doctor's salary? That for this salary certain goods and services are provided to the client—the prison? That in addition to traditional medical services, the deal also includes informal, unspoken agreements to mask the prison operations?

Revelations made during testimony before the U. S. Senate in 1968 and 1969 concerning general prison conditions in America strongly suggest that while the Arkansas prison conditions are probably more extensive in their depravity, they are by no means unique. Similar conditions have been reported in many jurisdictions, and it is conjectured that they exist in varying degrees in all 50 states.[6]

Most jails and all prisons provide some sort of medical services. They may be for emergency cases only, or may consist of a contractual relationship, a part-time or full-time physician, or, as in a few cases, there may be complete medical facilities within the prison complex. In terms of the arguments presented above, the layman can understand, if not accept, silence on matters of prison brutality by the individual doctors involved in these programs. The relationship between a physician and his prison-system client is confidential. But how can a collective silence by professional groups such as the American Medical Association be explained?

Is it possible that the medical profession is unaware of prison brutality? This contention seems unlikely, since the horrors of prison conditions are frequently reported by the media. Also, the thousands of doctors serving penal institutions presumably share their personal experiences at conferences. Yet, the silence continues. Is it possible that the profession has embraced the rationale of the individual physician and seeks to preserve the doctor (prison physician)-client (prison) relationship?

It is commendable that a profession has developed the expertise to transplant a human heart, to join severed body parts, and to create a rudimentary form of life. It is *condemnable* that this same profession tolerates stopping a human heart, severing body parts, and destruction of life.

Edmund Burke once observed that "the only thing necessary for the triumph of evil is for good men to do nothing, and remain silent." The members of the medical profession have been silent for too long. Humanitarian concepts dictate that the comfort, complacency, and sterile sanctity of "pure research" be relegated to a proper perspective and that commitments be made to eliminating such brutal conditions as those that exist in our prisons. The role of the prison physician, medical doctors in general, and especially the professional associations should be expanded to implement the tenets set forth in the Hippocratic Oath.

On February 13, 1968, Dr. Rodney F. Carlton, state pathologist of Arkansas, concluded from his examination of the three skeletons excavated at Cummins Prison that they did not show "any evidence of trauma or a violent death".[7] That is an interesting professional, medical opinion — especially in view of the fact that two of the bodies had been decapitated prior to burial and the skull of the third had been crushed to the size of a grapefruit.

Substantial evidence indicates that at least 200 more allegedly murdered inmates are still buried at Cummins Prison Farm. The three skeletons remain in the state pathologist's laboratory; the three excavations in the mule pasture have been filled; the inmates march silently to the fields each day and ponder the mystery of their being confined in a prison for "antisocial acts," while those chosen to "correct" them apparently condone murder under the mask of the law.

Is murder the exclusive domain of the legal profession and the criminal justice system, or does the medical profession have an ethical responsibility to deal with murder in a way compatible with its commitment to the sanctity of life?

References

1. Arkansas State Police, Criminal Investigations Division, *Case Report: Tucker State Prison Farm, Tucker, Arkansas*, (Little Rock: circa September, 1966).
2. *New York Times*, July 29, 1969, pp. 1, 20-21.
3. *Pine Bluff Commercial*, Pine Bluff, Arkansas March 29, 1967, p. 2.
4. Walter Rugaber, *New York Times, loc. cit.*
5. *Pine Bluff Commercial*, October 31, 1967, p. 1.
6. Inmate Danny Bennett died in a Mississippi state prison on June 17, 1970, of "heat stroke," according to prison physician Dr. B. L. Hammack. An autopsy later disclosed that Bennett died as the result of "a combination of both heat stroke and the results of severe trauma such as might have been [in]flicted in a beating." A legislative investigating committee found that Bennett "was murdered by one or more persons" and that the prison doctor either "knowingly misrepresented" the cause of death or was negligent or incompetent "to make a correct determination" (*The Delta Democrat-Times*, Greenville, Mississippi, January 20, 1971, p. 1).
7. *Arkansas Gazette*, February 13, 1968, p. 1.

CHAPTER 12

MEDICINE AND THE MILITARY

SOME ETHICAL PROBLEMS

Gordon S. Livingston

The regimen I adopt shall be for the benefit of my patients according to my ability and judgment, and not for their hurt or for any wrong.

—Hippocratic Oath

I will practice my profession with conscience and dignity; the health of my patient will be my first consideration.

—Declaration of Geneva (1948)

The principal objective of the medical profession is to render service to humanity with full respect for the dignity of man.

—Opinions and Reports of the
Judicial Council of the
American Medical Association (1966)

The Army Medical Service is a supporting service of the combat elements of the Army primarily concerned with the maintenance of the health and fighting efficiency of the troops....Its mission is to conserve manpower for early return to duty.

—U.S. Army Field Manual 8-10

In his laborious and checkered efforts to bring order and a sense of lasting value to his life, man has evolved and codified a multitude of behaviors. None of these efforts, even when cloaked in the mantle of divine sanction, has succeeded in eliminating the various forms of inhumanity which have resulted in the periodic murder of large numbers of human beings, and which now threaten the existence of all life on the planet.

Nowhere has the urge to codify behavior been more resolute than in the healing profession. The reasons for this are not wholly clear. Perhaps they include awe at confronting the mysteries and complexities of the human body and its processes, about which our ignorance has always been infinitely greater than our knowledge. Certainly there has always been a particular awareness of the fragility and evanescence of life and the terrible finality of death. Perhaps the codes grew out of a conviction that those who presumed to influence the lives of their fellows in such profound and potentially destructive ways undertook a special obligation to those whom they treated. This idea is expressed in the ancient Latin dictum "*primum non nocere*"—first, do no harm. Also, the high esteem which physicians have traditionally enjoyed seems to have imposed on them a special sense of obligation, even moral élitism.

Many rules of conduct have emerged over the centuries, some of them containing injunctions which sound archaic to the modern ear (e. g. the Hippocratic pledge to treat one's teachers as parents). But the distillation of the medical ethic, present in some form in each of the several codes, is a statement of obligation to the *individual* patient. The uniqueness of the physician's humane duty to his fellows found expression in his caring for them one at a time. This obligation was felt to transcend the doctor's allegiance to any particular political institution or philosophy, though they were by no means necessarily incompatible. Indeed, during the periodic collisions of competing political systems physicians have generally been awarded noncombatant status, and have been expected to do what they could to mitigate the suffering of those on both sides. The Declaration of Geneva contained the following pledge: "I will not permit considerations of religion, nationality, race, party, politics or social standing to intervene between my duty and my patient." All these attempts to define the behavior of those who practice the healing art, with its implied dedication to the individual, can perhaps be reduced to Lister's assertion: "The one rule of practice is to put yourself in the patient's place."

Theoretically, there is no inherent ethical conflict in the practice of medicine within the military, the physician being expected only to treat anyone who presents himself or is brought to him for care. In fact, however, organizational and individual needs are often incompatible: This is the ethical dilemma of the military physician. I would like to illustrate this from my own experience in a combat zone, for in war one views the military at its real work, where ethical subtleties resolve into the realities of life and death. And if the generalizations contained in any code of ethics are to have meaning it must be found in their specific application.

Unlike Americans wounded in Vietnam, who were flown directly to large evacuation hospitals with full surgical facilities, wounded Vietcong and North Vietnamese were brought to our regimental command post for questioning. It was my responsibility to give them what care I could with the very limited facilities at my disposal until the interrogation was completed. One night when I protested to my commanding officer that a wounded soldier might die if he were not promptly evacuated, I was told to "just keep him alive for a few minutes so we can question him. After that he can die; it doesn't matter to me."

I was confronted with several cases of "combat neurosis" who told me that they saw nothing in what they were doing that justified the risks they were being asked to take. In effect, they had seen enough of death to know that they preferred life. What was I to do with deviant behavior like that? They were given a brief respite and returned to their units; the fighting strength was conserved. How many were later killed I do not know, nor do I wish to.

On Christmas Eve, 1968, I was sitting down to supper at a surgical hospital when they brought in 33 Vietnamese children burned by the accidental explosion of a white phosphorus grenade. Some were blinded, some dying; all will carry the scars of that night for the rest of their lives, and, in a sense, so will I. That grenade, like so much of the misery in Vietnam, intentional and accidental, was made in U.S.A.

There was also the experience of working in the emergency room of an evacuation hospital and watching the MedEvac helicopters discharge their seemingly endless cargo of ruined lives. Here, as in the fields and villages of Vietnam, one saw the "product" of the huge technological combine which we have applied to the "problem" of this war. The wounded came in with tags affixed, and as we worked to salvage what we could, the proper functionary tried to obtain the data necessary for processing the "casualty." Words cannot convey the spectacle of a semiconscious man on a blood-soaked stretcher being asked to recall his social security number.

Then there is "Medical Civic Action," ostensibly directed toward helping the people of Vietnam. The concept is simple enough; U.S. medical personnel go out to a local village, set up shop, and provide treatment for anyone who needs it. The Vietnamese, of course, respond enthusiastically to this opportunity to receive the benefits of modern medical science, and flock to be treated. Unfortunately, treatment is limited by several circumstances: First, diagnosis is complicated by the difficulty of getting symptoms through an interpreter; diagnostic tools available include the stethoscope and the doctor's clinical acumen. Most important, however, is the complete inability to treat adequately any but the most superficial problems. Any given village is unlikely to be visited more often than every two months, if that, and official policy is to restrict distribution of medicines to a two-day supply lest excess fall to the Vietcong. The result of all this is a parody of medical care unsatisfying to both patients and physicians; most of the latter feel quite cynical about their role in this charade. One cannot treat obvious cases of tuberculosis with cough medicine and still retain a feeling of professional competence. This classic example of medicine as a political instrument was described by Brig. Gen. Spurgeon Neel, M.D., former Surgeon of the U.S. Military Assistance Command Vietnam, as a means of "maintaining the favorable image of the Central Government of Vietnam and of the U.S. in the minds of the general population."

And, finally, I ask you to consider a suggestion made to me by the Army's chief anesthesiologist in Vietnam—that we might induce prisoners to talk by using succinyl choline to paralyze the muscles of respiration. He offered to administer the drug.

It can be argued that the pressures of combat produce situations and behavior fundamentally different from those encountered during service in another time or place. Perhaps. But it seems clear to me that to the degree that the needs of the military are inherently inimical to the needs of those whom it uses, the physician who must deal with both is confronted with a divided loyalty, and the pressure to conform to the needs of the organization is nearly irresistible. An example is the use of psychiatric "diagnoses" to expedite the handling of behavior which the military considers deviant.

One Army psychiatrist who served in Vietnam published a paper describing the in-patient treatment of psychiatric casualties with high doses of tranquilizing drugs. He reported that this method enabled men with a wide variety of disorders to return to combat. The psychiatrist asserted that "such care neither oversimplifies issues nor encumbers and compromises the evaluation or treatment setting by intrusion of the psychiatrist's moral judgments and emotions." Commenting on this assertion another physician wrote, "It depends on what we mean by care. . .It is clear to me that giving a man 100 milligrams of Thorazine hourly by mouth until he is unconscious and maintaining him that way for 40 hours may be defined in another manner. Since it was given as a adjunct to a program to preserve fighting strength, we could call it 'persuasion' or 'helping one to face responsibility' or—less kindly—'coercion'. It takes semantic stretching to call it 'care.' "

Much has been written elsewhere about the excesses committed by our forces in Vietnam. No one can reasonably claim to be unaware that war crimes, as defined at Nuremberg and elsewhere, have occurred. In a sense we are all veterans of this war, numbed by long exposure to death and to the brutality that has always been a component of the combat experience. This situation presents a particular challenge to medicine, because the specific nature of the medical support required for the prosecution of the war conflicts with the traditionally humane values of the physician.

In its simplest terms, the ethical conflict implicit in military medicine is the confrontation between the individual and the organization which is certainly one of the fundamental issues of our times. We have all lost control of our lives. To one degree or another we are in the grip of giant bureaucracies which derive their power from a general acquiescence to their mandates. It is becoming more and more evident that the things produced, intentionally and incidentally, by these large organizations are not consistently useful or constructive. In fact, they have a depressing tendency to be things like dead bodies, a polluted environment, and, even for the fortunate, a steadily deteriorating quality of life. The military is merely one of the more evidently destructive contemporary bureaucracies. Like all the others, private and governmental, it functions by the efforts of those who serve it and those who accept the results.

Like the other institutions of a society, the practice of medicine generally reflects the dominant contemporary values. In the case of present-day America our worship of technology makes us think that the problems of our world, social and otherwise, are uniformly susceptible to the proper application of resources and good old American "know-how." The expedition to the moon was a classic example (and primary reinforcer) of this ethic. In Indochina the technological approach to social issues has failed us at an awesome cost, and, to a significant degree, medicine has been a willing adjunct to this massive misapplication of national power. At the very least one can state that without medical support the prosecution of this war would not have been possible. Individually and collectively, physicians have seen their skills employed by their government both to sanction and to perpetuate one of the most antilife enterprises of our time. What we have witnessed is the final distortion of our values, which could perhaps be expressed as an exercise in moral alchemy: To render evil into good it is only necessary to institutionalize it. Physicians have been persuaded to accept the organized murder of hundreds of thousands of human beings by being allowed (even required) to treat some of the survivors of the carnage, thus satisfying the medical impulse to serve while not examining the "political" assumptions and requirements which produced these results. It is perhaps worthwhile to recall here the statement of Karl Brandt concerning the German physicians who were convicted of crimes related to dangerous, often fatal, experimentation upon prisoners and mental defectives during World War II: "...it seems to be of small moment for the future whether the imposed code of contempt for the dignity of man issues from bureaucratic indifference or ideological aggression."

Argument is in progress within several professional organizations about whether physicians as a group should take positions on sociopolitical issues which are not generally considered to be within their field of expertise. The American Psychiatric Association has been divided on the question of whether to release the results of an opinion poll of its membership concerning the war. One of the more cogent arguments raised by those who oppose such release is a presumed threat to the tax-exempt status of the organization. It seems to me that if physicians are concerned with the effects of the social milieu on the lives of those whom they serve as individuals, they must come to grips with the questions affecting that milieu. Our cities are decaying, our people are divided, our children reject us and our values, turning in ever larger numbers to drugs and radicalism. Our spirits are numb with body-counts and destruction; we choke on our air; there is violence all about us. Medical research projects are closing down all over the country for lack of funding while we spend 70 billion dollars a year for "defense". And, amid all this, some of my colleagues fear that their professional organization might lose its tax-exempt status if the views of its membership were public knowledge. Medicine has come to this pass in its attempts to remain "apolitical." One notes in passing that the American College of Cardiology, without a trace of irony, gave its 1971 "Humanitarian of the Year" award to Richard Nixon.

It seems to me hopeless to argue that there have always been, and always will be, violence and war, and that physicians must be content to mitigate the effects. For something has changed in our lifetimes. The shadow of the final war hangs over us all, and to accept the inevitability of organized, armed human conflict is to accept, for ourselves and for our children, the prospect of the last death. Our business is with life. It is time we were about it.

CHAPTER 13

BEYOND ATROCITY

A PERSONAL PSYCHIATRIC VIEW

Robert Jay Lifton

***Introduction to Crimes of War, co-edited by Richard Falk, Gabriel Kolko, and Robert Jay Lifton**

The landscape doesn't change much. For days and days you see just about nothing. It's unfamiliar—always unfamiliar.Even when you go back to the same place, it's unfamiliar. And it makes you feel as though, well, there's nothing left in the world but this. . . . You have the illusion of going great distances and traveling, like hundreds of miles. . . .and you end up in the same place because you're only a couple of miles away. . . .But you feel like it's not all real. It couldn't possibly be. We couldn't still be in this country. We've been walking for days. . . .You're in Vietnam and they're using real bullets. . . .Here in Vietnam they're actually shooting people for no reason. . . Any other time you think, it's such an extreme. Here you can go ahead and shoot them for nothing. . . .As a matter of fact it's even. . .smiled upon, you know. Good for you. Everything is backwards. That's part of the kind of unreality of the thing. To the "grunt" [infantryman] this isn't backwards. He doesn't understand. . . .But something [at My Lai] was missing. Something you thought was real that would accompany this. It wasn't there. . . .There was something missing in the whole business that made it seem like it really wasn't happening. . . .

—American G.I.'s recollections of My Lai (personal interview)

When asked to speak at a number of recent occasions, I have announced my title as "On Living in Atrocity." To be sure neither I nor anyone else lives there all or even most of the time. But at this moment, in mid-1970, an American investigator of atrocity finds himself dealing with something that has become, for his countrymen in general, a terrible subterranean image that can neither be fully faced nor wished away. There is virtue in bringing that image to the surface.

In one sense, no matter what happens in the external world, personal atrocity, for everyone, begins at birth. It can also be said that some of us have a special nose for atrocity. Yet I can remember very well, during the early stirrings of the academic peace movement taking place around Harvard University during the mid and late 1950's—about 200 years ago, it now seems—how hard it was for us to feel what might happen at the other end of a nuclear weapon. Whatever one's nose for atrocities, there are difficulties surrounding the imaginative act of coming to grips with them.

After six months of living and working in Hiroshima, studying the human effects of the first atomic bomb, I found that these difficulties were partly overcome and partly exacerbated. On the one hand I learned all too well to feel what happened at the other end of an atomic bomb. But on the other hand I became impressed with the increasing gap we face between our technological capacity for perpetrating atrocities and our imaginative ability to confront their full actuality. Yet the attempt to narrow that gap can be enlightening, even liberating. For me Hiroshima was a profoundly "radicalizing" experience—not in any strict ideological sense but in terms of fundamental issues of living and dying, of how one lives, how one may die.

Whatever the contributing wartime pressures, Hiroshima looms as a paradigm of technological atrocity. Each of the major psychological themes of Hiroshima survivors—death immersion, psychic numbing, residual guilt—has direct relationship to its hideously cool and vast technological character. The specific technology of the bomb converted the brief moment of exposure into a lifelong encounter with death—through the sequence of the survivor's early immersion in massive and grotesque death and dying, is experiencing or witnessing bizarre and frequently fatal acute radiation effects during the following weeks and months, his knowledge of the increased incidence over the years of various forms (always fatal) of leukemia and cancer, and finally his acquisition of a death-tainted group identity, an "identity of the dead" or shared sense of feeling emotionally bound both to those killed by the bomb and to the continuing worldwide specter of nuclear genocide.

The experience of psychic numbing, or emotional desensitization—what some survivors called "paralysis of the mind"—was a necessary defense against feeling what they clearly knew to be happening. But when one looks further into the matter one discovers that those who made and planned the use of that first nuclear weapon—and those who today make its successors and plan their use—require their own form of psychic numbing. They too cannot afford to feel what they cognitively know would happen.

Victims and victimizers also shared a sense of guilt, expressed partly in a conspiracy of silence, a prolonged absence of any systematic attempt to learn about the combined physical and psychic assaults of the bomb on human beings. Survivors felt guilty about remaining alive while others died, and also experienced an amorphous sense of having been part of, having imbibed, the overall evil of the atrocity.The perpetrators of Hiroshima (and those in various ways associated with them)—American scientists, military and political leaders, and ordinary people—felt their own forms of guilt, though, ironically, in less tangible form than that of victims. Yet one cannot but wonder to what extent Hiroshima produced in Americans (and others) a guilt-associated sense that if we could do this we could do anything; and that anyone could do anything to us; in other words, an anticipatory sense of unlimited atrocity.

If these are lessons of Hiroshima, one has to learn them personally. My own immersion in massive death during investigations in that city, though much more privileged and infinitely less brutal, will nonetheless be as permanent as that of Hiroshima survivors themselves; as in their case it has profoundly changed my relationship to my own death as well as to all collective forms of death that stalk us. I had a similarly personal lesson regarding psychic numbing. During my first few interviews in Hiroshima I felt overwhelmed by the grotesque horrors described to me, but within the short space of a week or so this feeling gave way to a much more comfortable sense of myself as a psychological investigator, still deeply troubled by what he heard but undeterred from his investigative commitment. This kind of partial, task-oriented numbing now strikes me as inevitable and, in this situation, useful, yet at the same time potentially malignant in its implications.

By "becoming" a Hiroshima survivor (as anyone who opens himself to the experience must), while at the same time remaining an American, I shared something of both victim's and victimizer's sense of guilt. This kind of guilt by identification has its pitfalls, but I believe it to be one of the few genuine psychological avenues to confrontation of atrocity. For these three psychological themes are hardly confined to Hiroshima: Death immersion, psychic numbing, and guilt are a psychic trinity found in all atrocity.

Hiroshima also taught me the value and appropriateness of what I would call the apocalyptic imagination. The term offends our notions of steadiness and balance. But the technological dimensions of contemporary atrocity seem to me to require that we attune our imaginations to processes that are apocalyptic in the full dictionary meaning of the word—processes that are "wildly unrestrained" and "ultimately decisive," that involve "forecasting or predicting the ultimate destiny of the world in the shape of future events" and "foreboding imminent disaster of final doom."

In the past this kind of imagination has been viewed as no more than the "world-ending" delusion of the psychotic patient. But for the people of Hiroshima the "end of the world"—or something very close to it—became part of the actuality of their experience. Thus one survivor recalled: "My body seemed all black, everything seemed dark, dark all over. . .then I thought, 'The world is ending.' " And another: "The feeling I had was that everyone was dead. . . .I thought this was the end of Hiroshima—of Japan—of humankind." Those witnessing Nazi mass murder—the greatest of all man's atrocities to date—called forth similar images, though they could usually perceive that the annihilating process was in some way selective (affecting mainly Jews or anti-Nazis, or other specific groups). As Hiroshima took me to Auschwitz and Treblinka, however, I was struck mostly by the similarities and parallels in the overall psychology of atrocity.

Yet similar end-of-the-world impressions have been recorded in connection with "God-made" atrocities, as in the case of survivors' accounts of the plagues of the Middle Ages:

> How will posterity believe that there has been a time when without the lightings of heaven or the fires of earth, without wars or other visible slaughter, not this or that part of the earth, but well-nigh the whole globe, has remained without inhabitants. . . We should think we were dreaming if we did not with our eyes, when we walk abroad, see the city in mourning with funerals, and returning to our home, find it empty, and thus know that what we lament is real.

The plagues were God-made not only in the sense of being a mysterious and deadly form of illness outside of man's initiation or control but also because they could be comprehended as part of a God-centered cosmology. To be sure scenes like the above strained people's belief in an ordered universe and a just God, but their cosmology contained enough devils, enough flexibility, and enough depth of imprint to provide, if not a full "explanation" of holocaust, at least a continuing psychic framework within which to go on living. In contrast, Hiroshima and Auschwitz were initiated and carried out by men upon men, and at a time when old cosmologies had already lost much of their hold and could provide little explanatory power. Survivors were left with an overwhelming sense of dislocation and absurdity: Like the G.I. quoted earlier in relationship to My Lai, something for them was "missing"—namely, meaning or a sense of reality. With Hiroshima and Auschwitz now part of man's historical experience, it is dangerously naive to insist that our imaginative relationship to world-destruction can remain unchanged—that we can continue to make a simple-minded distinction between psychotic proclivity for, and "normal" avoidance of, that image.

Yet whatever the force of external events, there must be a subjective, imaginative component to the perceived "end of the world." Hiroshima survivors had to call forth early inner images of separation and helplessness, of stasis and annihilation, images available from everyone's infancy and childhood, but to some with greater force than to others. There is therefore a danger, not just for Hiroshima survivors but for all of us, of being trapped in such images, bound by a psychic sense of doom to the point of being immobilized and totally unable or unwilling to participate in essential day-by-day struggles to counter atrocity and prevent the collective annihilation imagined.

Psychological wisdom, then, seems to lie in neither wallowing in, nor numbing ourselves to, our imaginings of apocalypse. A simple example of the constructive use of the apocalyptic imagination is recorded by Eugene Rabinowitch, from the beginning an articulate leader in scientists' anti-atomic-bomb movements, Rabinowitch describes how, when walking down the streets of Chicago during the spring of 1945, he looked up at the city's great buildings and suddenly imagined a holocaust in which skyscrapers crumbled. He then vowed to redouble his efforts to prevent that kind of event from happening by means of the scientists' petition he and others were drawing up to head off the dropping of an atomic bomb, without warning, on a populated area. The effort of course failed, but this kind of apocalyptic imagination—on the part of Rabinowitch, Leo Szilard, and Bertrand Russell among others—has made it possible for at least a small minority of men and women to name and face the true conditions of our existence.* For we live in the shadow of the ultimate atrocity, of the potentially terminal revolution—and if that term is itself a contradiction, the same contradiction is the central fact of our relationship to death and life.

We perpetrate and experience the American atrocity at My Lai in the context of these apocalyptic absurdities and dislocations. The G.I.'s quoted description suggests not only that atrocity can be a dreamlike affair (in this sense, resembling the quoted passage about the place), but that it is committed by men living outside of ordinary human connection, outside of both society and history. My Lai was acted out by men who had lost their bearings, men wandering about in both a military and psychic no-man's land. The atrocity itself can be seen as a grotesquely paradoxical effort to put straight this crooked landscape, to find order and significance in disorder and absurdity. There is at the same time an impulse to carry existing absurdity and disorder to their logical extreme, as if both to transcend and demonstrate that aberrant existential state.

Atrocities are committed by desperate men—in the case of My Lai, men victimized by the absolute contradictions of the war they were asked to fight, by the murderous illusions of their country's policy. Atrocity, then, is a perverse quest for meaning, the end result of a spurious sense of mission, the product of false witness.

To say that American military involvement in Vietnam is itself a crime is also to say that it is an atrocity-producing situation. Or to put the matter another way, My Lai illuminates, as nothing else has, the essential nature of America's war in Vietnam. The elements of this atrocity-producing situation include an advanced industrial nation engaged in a counterinsurgency action in an underdeveloped area, against guerrillas who merge with the people—precisely the elements which Jean-Paul Sartre has described as inevitably genocidal. In the starkness of its murders and the extreme dehumanization experienced by victimizers and imposed on victims, My Lai reveals to us how far America has gone along the path of deadly illusion.

Associated with this deadly illusion are three psychological patterns as painful to the sensitized American critic of the war as they are self-evident. The first is the principle of atrocity building upon atrocity, because of the need to deny the atrocity-producing situation. In this sense My Lai itself was a product of earlier, smaller My Lais; and it was followed not by an ending of the war but by the American extension of the war into Laos and Cambodia.

The second principle involves the system of nonresponsibility. One searches in vain for a man or group of men who will come forward to take the blame or even identify a human source of responsibility for what took place: from those who fired the bullets at My Lai (who must bear some responsibility, but were essentially pawns and victims of the atrocity-producing situation, and are now being made scapegoats as well); to the junior-grade officers who gave orders to do the firing and apparently did some of it themselves; to the senior-grade officers who seemed to have ordered the operation; to the highest military and civilian planners in Vietnam, the Pentagon, and the White House who set such policies as that of a "*permanent* free-fire zone" (which, according to Richard Hammer, means "in essence. . .that any Americans operating within it had, basically, a license to kill and any Vietnamese living within it had a license to be killed") and made even more basic decisions about continuing and even extending the war; to the amorphous conglomerate of the American people who, presumably, chose, or at least now tolerate, the aforementioned as their representatives. The atrocity-producing situation, at least in this case, depends upon what Masao Maruyama has called a "system of nonresponsibility." Situation and system alike are characterized by a technology and a technicized bureaucracy unchecked by sensate human minds.

The third and perhaps most terrible pattern is the psychology of nothing happening. General Westmoreland gives way to General Abrams, President Johnson to President Nixon, a visibly angry student generation to one silent with rage—and the war, the atrocity-producing situation, continues to grind out its thousands of recorded and unrecorded atrocities. To be more accurate, something does happen—the subliminal American perception of atrocity edges toward consciousness—making it more difficult but, unfortunately, not impossible to defend and maintain the atrocity-producing situation. The widespread feeling of being stuck in atrocity contributes, in ways we can now hardly grasp, to a national sense of degradation and a related attraction to violence. For nothing is more conducive to collective rage and totalism than a sense of being bound to a situation perceived to be both suffocating and evil.

Atrocity in general, and My Lai in particular, brings its perpetrators—even a whole nation—into the realm of existential evil. That state is exemplified by what another G.I. described to me as a working definition of the enemy in Vietnam: "If it's dead, it's VC—because it's dead. If it's dead, it *had* to be VC. And of course, a corpse couldn't defend itself anyhow." When at some future moment, ethically sensitive historians get around to telling the story of the Vietnam War—assuming that there will be ethically sensitive (or for that matter, any) historians around—I have no doubt that they will select the phenomenon of the "body count" as the perfect symbol of America's descent into evil. What better represents the numbing, brutalization, illusion (most of the bodies, after all, turn out to be those of civilians), grotesque competition (companies and individuals vie for the highest body counts), and equally grotesque technicizing (progress lies in the *count*) characteristic of the overall American crime of war in Vietnam.

My Lai is rather unusual in one respect. It combines two kinds of atrocity: technological overkill (of unarmed peasants by Americans using automatic weapons), and a more personal, face-to-face gunning-down of victims at point-blank range. This combination lends the incident particular psychic force, however Americans may try to fend off awareness of its implications. A participating G.I. could characterize My Lai as "just like a Nazi-type thing" (as recorded in Seymour Hersh's book, *My Lai 4*), a characterization made by few if any pilots or crewmen participating in the more technologically distanced killings of larger numbers of Vietnamese civilians from the air.

The sense of being associated with existential evil is new to Americans. This is so partly because such perceptions have been suppressed in other atrocity-producing situations, but also because of the humane elements of American tradition that contribute to a national self-image of opposing, through use of force if necessary, just this kind of "Nazi-type thing." The full effects of the war in Vietnam upon this self-image are at this point unclear. The returns from My Lai are not yet in. Perhaps they never are for atrocity. But I for one worry about a society that seems to absorb, with some questioning but without fundamental self-examination, first Hiroshima and now My Lai.

For there is always a cost. Atrocities have a way of coming home. The killings by National Guardsmen of Kent State students protesting the extension of the war in Cambodia reflect the use of violence in defense of illusion and denial of evil—and the killings of blacks at Augusta, Georgia and of black students at Jackson State in Mississippi reflect more indirectly that atmosphere. Indeed there is a real danger that the impulse to preserve illusion and deny evil could carry America beyond Vietnam and Cambodia into some form of world-destroying nuclear confrontation. In this sense, as well as in its relationship to existential evil, My Lai symbolized a shaking of the American foundations—a bitterly mocking perversion of what was left of the American dream. Like Hiroshima and Auschwitz, My Lai is a revolutionary event: Its total inversion of moral standards raises fundamental questions about the institutions and national practices of the nation responsible for it.

The problem facing Americans now is, What do we do with our atrocities? Do we simply try our best to absorb them by a kind of half-admission which denies their implications and prevents genuine confrontation? That is the classical method of governments for dealing with documented atrocities, and it is clearly the method being used by the United States government and military now in its legal trials of individuals. Those who did the shooting and those who covered up the event are being labeled aberrant and negligent, so that the larger truth of the atrocity-producing situation can be avoided. The award of a Pulitzer Prize to Seymour Hersh for his journalistic feat in uncovering the story of My Lai and telling it in detail would seem to be a step in the direction of that larger truth. Yet one cannot but fear that such an award—as in the case of the National Book Award I received for my work on Hiroshima—can serve as a form of conscience-salving taken recognition in place of confrontation. Surely more must be faced throughout American society, more must be articulated and given form by leaders and ordinary people, if this atrocity is to contribute to a national process of illumination instead of merely one of further degradation.

I am struck by how little my own profession has had to say about the matter—about the way in which aberrant *situations* can produce collective disturbance and mass murder. The psychiatry and psychohistory I would like to envisage for the future would put such matters at its center. It would also encourage combining ethical involvement with professional skills in ways that could simultaneously shed light upon such crimes of war and contribute to the transformation our country so desperately requires. In dealing with our dislocations we

need to replace the false witness of atrocity with the genuine witness of new and liberating forms and directions. The task, then, is to confront atrocity in order to move beyond it.

NOTE

1. Bertrand Russell had earlier exhibited the dangers of the apocalyptic imagination when he advocated that we threaten to drop atomic bombs on Russia in order to compel her to agree to a system of international control of nuclear weapons.

CHAPTER 14

SOCIAL ETHICS FOR MEDICAL EDUCATORS

John G. Bruhn and Douglas C. Smith

Dobzhansky[1] has commented, "By changing what he knows about the world, man changes the world he knows; and by changing the world in which he lives, man changes himself." Man has changed medicine; medicine has changed man; and together they have changed the world. These interlocking changes have not occurred in orderly transition. Often a medical breakthrough has resulted in a problem-laden gap. For example, man's longevity has been increased through the discovery of lifesaving techniques and greater knowledge about the etiology and treatment of disease; but increased longevity has deepened and complicated the interrelationships between the patterning of disease and man's way of life. Furthermore this or any new knowledge may prove to be more detrimental than beneficial unless medical educators, as well as practitioners and researchers are willing to face the evolving triad—knowledge, practice and social responsibility. As Dubos[2] has observed, the diseases of greatest prevalence are the diseases of scarcity and the diseases of civilization.

Despite the rapid and pervasive effects of social change on other institutions, medicine has maintained that its first responsibility is to care for patients in hospitals and offices. The power, politics and organization of medicine have resisted an expansion of the social responsibility of physicians to areas of community life removed from direct patient care. In a convocation address in 1965, Dr. Ivan Bennett said: "... the inclination of many doctors to obstruct social change tends to make them strangers to the public and to colleagues with a greater social conscience."[3] Yet at the same time the mass media have familiarized the public with health care knowledge and its potentials. As the gap widens between the changing health needs of the public and the narrow view of social responsibility in medicine, public pressure has mounted to directly challenge medicine's response to our health-care crisis.

There are insufficient numbers of physicians to meet the increasing health needs of the public, but educating more physicians alone will not meet current health needs.[4] What is essential is the training of physicians and allied health professionals who are committed to delivering health care in the community. While the concept of medical care as a right may have been accepted in principle by both the public and medicine, health professionals have not developed a system capable of granting that right.

The concept of social responsibility must permeate our system of medical education if such a system is to be developed. Clinical responsibility is traditionally a highly valued attribute of the physician; the ability to assume and delegate it is considered the ultimate foundation of clinical maturity. Social responsibility, however, has been narrowly conceived and usually left to the realm of experience or chance; it is something the student will develop or "pick up" as he progresses through medical school. The faculty reinforce this concept of social responsibility by relegating it to the "art" of medicine.[5]

Some medical schools have altered their curricula in varying degrees in an attempt to expose students to the relationships between human behavior and health or disease. Some of these changes include establishing courses in the social sciences and humanities, introducing patients to students from the onset of medical school, providing more time for electives which can be taken within the university at large, and integrating basic science and clinical phenomena in a "systems approach" to health and disease. Courses in "Man and His Environment" are now common, but few involve physicians except for occasional lectures, and seldom does the course extend beyond the preclinical years. Frequently revisions in the medical school curriculum have amounted to little more than the juggling of class hours, renaming of courses, and forced "interdisciplinary" teaching alliances between departments as a result of cuts in the teaching hours of some basic science courses. Little progress has been made in deciding what kind of product medical schools need to turn out in order to deliver health care more effectively in a changing society.

Little has been done to alter premedical training: hence, students applying to medical schools are encouraged to gear their baccalaureate education toward the biological and physical sciences. Students learn the "system" for applying to medical school. Their outward appearance may be temporarily altered for the admission interview, while their ideas, values and beliefs remain hidden—much to the chagrin of the committee. Some students, who are more vocal about their beliefs and values, however, have not been dissuaded from applying. A recent study reports that the characteristics of politically active students in college are consistent with those of social-activist groups in medical schools. The report states, "Such evidence would suggest that we are now observing the first cohort of students who were 'turned on' before matriculation to medical school. If so, then medical educators and practitioners may anticipate not a single wave or epidemic of activists, but that the phonomenon will become endemic, barring the institution of quarantine procedures by admission committees."[6] Students have provided, and undoubtedly will continue to provide, much of the impetus for change in premedical and medical curricula. Students attempts at change have, for the most part, been orderly, constructive, and persistent in formulating challenging learning experiences in medical school and in the community.

One modern complaint about medical education is that it is too rigid, designed to mold specialists. By the same token it would be erroneous to redesign the curriculum to mold only generalists or community-oriented physicians, for our medical care system needs both. There should, however, be flexibility enough to permit the latter type to develop without stigmatization by faculty and students. The need to specialize in order to treat "the whole person" is paradoxical; nonetheless, specialization and subspecialization are held out as the ultimate rewards of medical achievement, and even family medicine has succumbed to the need for specialty status. The hope of abating future mass migration to the specialties lies in part in permitting future physicians to see and learn about societal health needs, and to experience the gratifications of providing care beyond the rewards of status, prestige, and money. This necessitates a revamping of the route to becoming a physician. Present requirements permit little time for students to obtain more than a passing acquaintance with the behavioral science and humanities majors are implicitly or explicitly discouraged from applying to medical school. Admission criteria should include a more balanced assessment of knowledge, ability, and professional promise.

All medical students should be exposed to the principles and concepts of human behavior as these relate to health as well as to disease. Moreover, this material should be integrated with teaching and clinical experience throughout medical school. Students should be encouraged to take electives in medical ethics, medical economics, health administration, social issues in medicine, genetic counseling, family planning, health education, behavioral science, and so forth. New knowledge has shaped new definitions of disease. Zilboorg[7] points out that "general medicine never has to ask itself what disease is—it always knew what it meant to be ill and both the patient and doctor knew what pain and other forms of physical suffering were." Social well-being, mental health, and psychological normality, on the other hand, are not clearly defined, and notions about them vary greatly in different sociological and historical circumstances.[8] Since physical, social, and emotional well-being are intricately related, changing social definitions of well-being must, in turn, influence physical definitions. Thus it is appropriate to question the efficacy of a disease-free state. We have persisted in viewing health as the absence of disease, and this illusion of absolute normality has ignored the possibility that "the right amount of disease at the right time" might facilitate social and/or psychological adaptation. The possibility that illness can be a socially acceptable and effective response in coping with life situations further challenges the efficacy of the alleviation of all pain as a basic premise of medical treatment. Indeed, in some individuals analgesics may inhibit social adaptation more than the persistence of unalleviated pain.

Dixon has suggested that one way to teach physicians to become agents of social change is for medical schools to become involved in the direct provision of health services in poor and rural areas where neglect abounds.[9] Faculty and students must experience first hand the ineptness of the current conventional methods of health care delivery. Only direct involvement with the powerless inhabitants of a world that lacks economic, social, political, and legal resources can imprint upon faculty and students alike the need for sweeping changes in our health care system. As Michaelson has suggested, "abuses will be uncovered first where they are most naked—among the poor and nonwhite—and at last where they are most subtle . . . among us all."[10] Our health-care system is not only élitist, but also deficient in quality. A physician usually evaluates the quality of health care in terms of the treatment given to an individual patient or part of his anatomy. Many health professionals are reluctant to accept the medical importance of social and psychological aspects of the patient's life.[11] Apparently, they either do not know or are indifferent to how often the recovery of health depends on the presence or absence of social support, hope, or life satisfaction. The challenge to medicine now is to frame a new set of goals and ethics in tune with current human needs. Only after goals have been established is it feasible to redesign a system for meeting these goals. Many solutions to our health-care crisis have been proposed, but none will succeed without the accompaniment of vast social developments.[12] Indeed, if health is a right there must be a system of maintenance and care flexible enough to adapt to its changing social parameters.

Physicians and medical educators must also address themselves to new responsibilities to mankind. Medicine's social responsibilities in a changing world also carry with them obligations to provide guidance in transforming social values. Greater control over life and death has increased the complexity of decisions physicians have had to make regarding the prolongation and termination of life. Biological technology has created a set of new social, political, and legal questions. Reducing infant mortality and prolonging life might be questioned as high-priority goals in the face of ecological warnings of overpopulation, hunger, and declining quality of life. A gradual transformation of social values has already become apparent in public attitudes toward human intervention at the beginning and end of life. Contraception and abortion are more accepted. Suicide and euthanasia are debated in public. A greater role is being demanded of health professionals in genetic counseling, family planning, and sex education. Preparation for these roles must not be left to chance.

The personal ethics involved in transactions between physicians and their individual patients are but one part of the total human situation, and cannot be divorced from the values held by society. Thus, the physician's social responsibility transcends responsibility for the individual patient. Increasingly medicine will be asked to assume a position of leadership in the re-examination of social values. An essential part of this leadership role is that of the teacher-practitioner who is an advocate for health education. Indeed, it will become increasingly necessary for the physician to teach patients how to prevent disease rather than only warn them about the consequences of their habits. As Freidson has pointed out, "by virtue of its occupational perspective, medicine always looks for and sees more illness than the lay world . . . and the process of treatment and care leads the patient to behave in the ways appropriate to the illness which has been diagnosed."[13] It should also be medicine's responsibility to recognize health and to assist patients in maintaining it.

In redesigning a system of health care as a right, medical educators as well as physicians have a social responsibility to apply scientific knowledge to human affairs. As old traditions in medicine have become ineffective in meeting new societal needs, there is little room for doubt that comprehensive health care should be the primary goal of contemporary medicine. "There is a need. . . for a new personal ethic for doctors and medical scientists. The Hippocratic Oath, noble in its intention, no longer serves. It has been overtaken by events."[14]

REFERENCES

1. T. Dobzhansky, *Mankind Evolving: The Evolution of the Human* Species (New Haven: Yale University Press, 1962).

2. R. Dubos, *Reason Awake* (New York: Columbia University Press, 1970).

3. L. Lasagna, *Life, Death and the Doctor* (New York: Alfred Knopf, 1968).

4. *The Graduate Education of Physicians,* Report of the Citizens Commission on Graduate Medical Education, American Medical Association (August, 1966).

5. J. G. Bruhn, "On Social Responsibility," *Journal of Medical* Education, 46 (1971), pp. 166-168.

6. C. E. Lewis, "A Longitudinal Study of Potential Change Agents in Medicine—A Preliminary Report," *Journal of Medical Education,* 44 (1969), pp. 1029-1034.

7. G. Zilboorg, *History of Medical Psychology* (New York: Norton, 1941).

8. F. J. Hacker, "The Concept of Normality and Its Practical Significance," *American Journal of Orthopsychiatry,* 15 (1945), pp. 47-64.

9. J. P. Dixon, "Teaching Physicians To Be Agents of Social Change," *Archives of Environmental Health,* 10 (1965), pp. 713-718.

10. M. G. Michaelson, "The Failure of Medicine," *American Scholar,* 39 (1970), pp. 694-706.

11. R. S. Duff and A. B. Hollingshead, *Sickness and Society* (New York: Harper and Row, 1968).

12. M. I. Roemer, "Nationalized Medicine," *Trans*-action, 8 (1971), pp. 31-36.

13. E. Freidson, *The Profession of Medicine* (New York: Dodd, Mead, 1970).

14. Lord Ritchie-Calder, "The Doctor's Dilemma," *The Center* Magazine, 4 (1971), pp. 71-75.

NOTES ABOUT THE CONTRIBUTORS

Walter C. Alvarez, Professor of Medicine Emeritus, University of Minnesota, and Senior Consultant Emeritus to Mayo Clinic, Rochester, Minnesota.

Leroy Augenstein, Deceased. Formerly Professor of Biophysics at Michigan State University, East Lansing, Michigan.

John G. Bruhn, Professor and Chairman, Department of Human Ecology, University of Oklahoma Medical Center.

Carleton B. Chapman, Dean and Professor of Medicine, Dartmouth Medical School.

H. Roy Kaplan, Assistant Professor of Sociology, State University of New York at Buffalo.

Marvin Kohl, Associate Professor of Philosophy, State University College, Fredonia, New York.

Louis Lasagna, Chairman, Department of Pharmacology and Toxicology, The University of Rochester School of Medicine and Dentistry, Rochester, New York.

Chauncey D. Leake, Professor of Medical Jurisprudence, Hastings College of Law. Formerly Professor, Department of Pharmacology, School of Medicine, University of California and Ohio State University, and Executive Vice-President for the Medical Branch, University of Texas.

Robert Jay Lifton, Foundations' Fund Research Professor of Psychiatry, Yale University. Former U.S. Air Force Medical Officer.

Gordon Livingston, Resident Physician in Psychiatry, John Hopkins. Formerly Regimental Surgeon, 11th Armored Cavalry Regiment. Resigned July 1969.

Tom Murton, Professor in the Department of Criminal Justice Studies, University of Minnesota. Formerly Warden of the Cummins Prison Farm in the State of Arkansas.

Patrick Romanell, H.Y. Benedict Professor of Philosophy, The University of Texas, El Paso.

Deborah Silverman, Background in Philosophy.

Mervyn F. Silverman, Director of Office for Consumer Affairs, Food and Drug Administration, Department of Health, Education and Welfare.

Douglas C. Smith, Medical Student, University of Oklahoma.

John M. Talmadge, Ziegler Foundation Fellow at Dartmouth in 1969-70. Presently enrolled in the Duke University School of Medicine.

Howard C. Taylor, Director of International Institute for the Study of Human Reproduction, and Rappleye Professor Emeritus of Obstetrics and Gynecology at the College of Physicians & Surgeons of Columbia University, New York City.

Maurice B. Visscher, Distinguished Service and Regents' Professor Emeritus, University of Minnesota.